Immunology at a Glance

STANDARD LOAN

UNLESS RECALLED BY ANOTHER READER
THIS ITEM MAY BE BORROWED FOR

FOUR WEEKS

To renew, telephone:
01243 816089 (Bishop Otter)
01243 816099 (Bognor Regis)

Immunology at a Glance

J.H.L. PLAYFAIR
Professor of Immunology
University College and Middlesex
School of Medicine
London

FIFTH EDITION

OXFORD
BLACKWELL SCIENTIFIC PUBLICATIONS
LONDON EDINBURGH BOSTON
MELBOURNE PARIS BERLIN VIENNA

First published 1979
Reprinted 1980
Italian edition 1981
Second edition 1982
Reprinted 1983 (twice)
Spanish edition 1983
Third edition 1984
Fourth edition 1987
Reprinted 1988, 1990, 1991
Japanese edition 1987
Fifth edition 1992
Reprinted 1992, 1993
Four Dragons edition 1992
Reprinted 1992, 1993

Set by Semantic Graphics, Singapore
Printed and bound in Great Britain
at the University Press, Cambridge

DISTRIBUTORS

Marston Book Services Ltd
PO Box 87
Oxford OX2 0DT
(*Orders*: Tel: 0865 791155
          Fax: 0865 791927
          Telex: 837515)

USA
Blackwell Scientific Publications, Inc.
238 Main Street
Cambridge, MA 02142
(*Orders*: Tel: 800 759-6102
          617 876-7000)

Canada
Times Mirror Professional Publishing Ltd.
130 Flaska Drive
Markham, Ontario L6G 1B8
(*Orders*: Tel: 800 268-4178
          416 470-6739)

Australia
Blackwell Scientific Publications Pty Ltd
54 University Street
Carlton, Victoria 3053
(*Orders*: Tel: 03 347-5552)

A catalogue record for this book is
available from the British Library.

ISBN 0-632-03315-0 (BSP)
ISBN 0-632-03377-0 (Four Dragons)

Contents

Immunity

1   The scope of immunology

2   Natural and adaptive immune mechanisms

3   Evolution of immune mechanisms

4   Cells involved in immunity: the haemopoietic system

Natural immunity

5   Complement

6   Acute inflammation

7   Phagocytic cells: the reticulo-endothelial system

8   Phagocytosis

Adaptive immunity

(i)   *The cellular basis*

9   Lymphocytes

10   Primary lymphoid organs and lymphopoiesis

11   Secondary lymphoid organs and lymphocyte traffic

(ii)   *The molecular basis*

12   Evolution of recognition molecules

13   The major histocompatibility complex

14   The T cell receptor

15   Antibody diversification and synthesis

16   Antibody structure and function

(iii)   *The adaptive immune response*

17   The antibody response

18   Antigen–antibody interaction and immune complexes

19   Cell-mediated immune responses

(iv)   *Regulation*

20   Tolerance

21   Idiotypes, anti-idiotypes and networks

22   The cytokine network

23   Immunity, hormones and the brain

Potentially useful immunity

24   Anti-microbial immunity: a general scheme

25   Immunity to bacteria

26   Immunity to viruses

27   Immunity to protozoa

28   Immunity to worms

29   Immunity to fungi

30   Immunity to tumours

Undesirable effects of immunity

31   Harmful immunity: a general scheme

32   Anaphylaxis and allergy

33   Immune complexes, complement and disease

34   Chronic and cell-mediated inflammation

35   Autoimmunity

36   Transplant rejection

Altered immunity

37   Immunosuppression

38   Immunodeficiency

39   HIV and AIDS

40   Immunostimulation and vaccination

Appendixes

41   Comparative sizes
Comparative molecular weights

42   Landmarks in the history of immunology
Some unsolved problems

43   The CD classification

Index

Preface

This is not a textbook for immunologists, who already have plenty of excellent ones to choose from. Rather, it is aimed at all those whose work immunology impinges on, but who may hitherto have lacked the time to keep abreast of a subject that can sometimes seem impossibly fast-moving and intricate.

Yet everyone with a background in medicine or the biological sciences is already familiar with a good deal of the basic knowledge required to understand immunological processes, often needing no more than a few quick blackboard sketches to see roughly how they work. This is a book of sketches which have proved useful over the years, recollected (and artistically touched up) in tranquillity.

The Chinese sage who remarked that one picture was worth a thousand words was certainly not an immunology teacher, or his estimate would not have been so low! In this book the text has been pruned to the minimum necessary for understanding the figures, omitting almost all historical and technical details, which can be found in the larger textbooks listed on the next page. In trying to steer a middle course between absolute clarity and absolute up-to-dateness, I am well aware of having missed both by a comfortable margin. But even in immunology, what is brand-new does not always turn out to be right, while the idea that any form of presentation, however unorthodox, will make simple what other authors have already shown to be complex can only be, in Dr Johnson's heartfelt words, 'the dream of a philosopher doomed to wake a lexicographer'. My object has merely been to convince workers in neighbouring fields that modern immunology is not quite as forbidding as they may have thought.

It is perhaps the price of specialization that some important aspects of nature lie between disciplines and are consequently ignored for many years (transplant rejection is a good example). It follows that scientists are wise to keep an eye on each others' areas so that in due course the appropriate new disciplines can emerge—as immunology itself did from the shared interests of bacteriologists, haematologists, chemists, and the rest.

Acknowledgements

My largest debt is obviously to the immunologists who made the discoveries this book is based on; if I had credited them all by name it would not have been a slim volume. In addition, I am grateful to my colleagues at the Middlesex Hospital for information, advice and criticism at all stages, particularly Dr J. Brostoff, Dr A. Cooke, Dr V. Eisen, Dr F.C. Hay, Dr P. Lydyard, Dr D. Male, Dr S. Marshall-Clarke and Professor I.M. Roitt. My secretary, Miss S. Bunce, and Mr R.R. Phillips and his colleagues in the photographic department of the Middlesex Hospital, worked tirelessly to get the manuscript and the figures right. I then showed the original draft to Professor H.E.M. Kay, Professor C.A. Mims and Professor L. Wolpert, all of whom made valuable suggestions for improvement. My son Edward supplied a useful undergraduate view. Finally I would like to thank Per Saugman of Blackwell Scientific Publications for his encouragement in the first place.

Note on the fifth edition

Little has changed radically in immunology since the last edition 5 years ago, but research on cytokines has accelerated to the point where they need a section of their own. I have included a section on the new field of psychoneuroimmunology, not because it is universally accepted but because it has aroused such a lot of interest—both professional and public. For the same reason I felt it was no longer possible to consider AIDS as just another viral disease, so that too has its own section now. Otherwise it has mainly been a question of updating terminology; there is a new appendix listing the now-routine CD names for cell surface molecules.

How to use this book

Each of the figures (listed in the contents) represents a particular topic, corresponding roughly to a 45-minute lecture. Newcomers to the subject may like first to read through the **text** (left-hand pages), using the figures only as a guide; this can be done at a sitting.

Once the general outline has been grasped, it is probably better to concentrate on the **figures** one at a a time. Some of them are quite complicated and can certainly not be taken in 'at a glance', but will need to be worked through with the help of the **legends** (right-hand pages), consulting the **index** for further information on individual details; once this has been done carefully they should subsequently require little more than a cursory look to refresh the memory.

It will be evident that the figures are highly diagrammatic and not to scale; indeed the scale often changes several times within one figure. For an idea of the actual sizes of some of the cells and molecules mentioned, refer to **Appendix 1** (Section 41).

The reader will also notice that examples are drawn sometimes from the mouse, in which useful animal so much fundamental immunology has been worked out, and sometimes from the human, which is after all the one that matters to most people. Luckily the two species are, from the immunologist's viewpoint, remarkably similar.

Further reading

I cannot do better than recommend the textbooks I myself consult regularly, and which largely furnished the raw material for this book.

Holborow E.J. & Reeves W.G. (eds) (1983) *Immunology in Medicine*, 2nd edn. Grune & Stratton, London (676 pp).

Hood L.E., Weissman I.L., Wood W.B. & Wilson J.H. (1984) *Immunology*, 2nd edn. The Benjamin/Cummings Publishing Co. Inc., California (558 pp).

Lachmann P.J. & Peters D.K. (eds) (1982) *Clinical Aspects of Immunology*, 4th edn. Blackwell Scientific Publications, Oxford (1751 pp).

McConnell I., Munro A. & Waldman H. (1981) *The Immune System*, 2nd edn. Blackwell Scientific Publications, Oxford (352 pp).

Mims C.A. (1987) *The Pathogenesis of Infectious Disease*, 3rd edn. Academic Press, London (342 pp).

Park B.H. & Good R.A. (1974) *Principles of Modern Immunobiology*. Lea & Febiger, Philadelphia (617 pp).

Roitt I.M. (1991) *Essential Immunology*, 7th edn. Blackwell Scientific Publications, Oxford (356 pp).

Roitt I.M., Brostoff J. & Male D.K. (1989) *Immunology*, 2nd edn. Churchill Livingstone, Gower, London (298 pp).

Stites D.P. & Tew A.I. (eds) (1991) *Basic and Clinical Immunology*, 7th edn. Lange Medical Publications, E. Norfolk, Connecticut (870 pp).

Thaler M.S., Klausner R.D. & Cohen H.J. (1977) *Medical Immunology*. J.B. Lippincott Co., Philadelphia (480 pp).

Weir D.M. (1977) *Immunology*. Churchill Livingstone, Edinburgh (206 pp).

Woolf N. (1986) *Cell, Tissue and Disease*, 2nd edn. Baillière Tindall, London (503 pp).

1 The scope of immunology

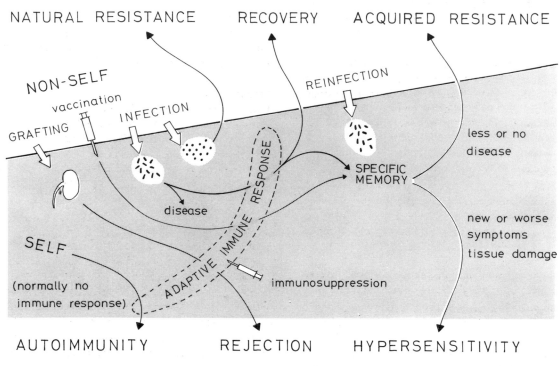

DESIRABLE CONSEQUENCES OF IMMUNITY

NATURAL RESISTANCE   RECOVERY   ACQUIRED RESISTANCE

UNDESIRABLE CONSEQUENCES OF IMMUNITY

AUTOIMMUNITY   REJECTION   HYPERSENSITIVITY

Of the four major causes of death—injury, infection, degenerative disease and cancer—only the first two regularly kill their victims before child-bearing age, which means that they are a potential source of lost genes. Therefore any mechanism that reduces their effects has tremendous survival value, and we see this in the processes of, respectively, **healing** and **immunity**.

Immunity is concerned with the recognition and disposal of foreign or 'non-self' material that enters the body (represented by white arrows in the figure), usually in the form of life-threatening infectious micro-organisms but sometimes, unfortunately, in the shape of a life-saving kidney graft. Resistance to infection may be **'natural'** (i.e. inborn and unchanging) or **'acquired'** as the result of an **adaptive immune response** (centre).

Immunology is the study of the organs, cells, and molecules responsible for this recognition and disposal (the 'immune system'), of how they respond and interact, of the consequences—desirable (top) or otherwise (bottom)—of their activity, and of the ways in which they can be advantageously increased or reduced.

Note that some scientists (e.g. Soviet) extend immunology to include other relationships between cells, for instance during embryonic development, at which most Western immunologists draw the line. Nature, presumably, is not prejudiced as to which type of specialist unveils her secrets, but the more restricted approach does so far seem to have led to more rapid progress. However, it is hard to imagine that in the long run immunologists and embryologists will not join forces, **recognition** being central to both disciplines.

Non-self

A widely used term in immunology, covering everything which is detectably different from an animal's own constituents. Infectious micro-organisms, together with cells, organs, or other materials from another animal, are the most important non-self substances from an immunological viewpoint, but drugs and even normal foods which are, of course, non-self too, can sometimes give rise to immunity.

Infection

Parasitic viruses, bacteria, protozoa, worms or fungi that attempt to gain access to the body or its surfaces are probably the chief *raison d'être* of the immune system. Higher animals whose immune system is damaged or deficient frequently succumb to infections which normal animals overcome.

Natural resistance

Entry of many micro-organisms (shown in the figure as black dots) is prevented, or they are rapidly eliminated, by antimicrobial defence mechanisms. Others (shown as black rods) can avoid elimination and survive to cause disease.

Adaptive immune response

The development or augmentation of defence mechanisms in response to a particular ('specific') stimulus, e.g. an infectious organism. It can result in elimination of the micro-organism and **recovery** from disease, and often leaves the host with **specific memory**, enabling it to respond more effectively on reinfection with the same micro-organism, a condition called **acquired resistance**. Since the body has no prior way of knowing which micro-organisms are harmless and which are not, all foreign material is usually responded to as if it were harmful, including relatively inoffensive pollens, etc.

Vaccination

A method of stimulating the adaptive immune response and generating memory and acquired resistance without suffering the full effects of the disease. The name comes from *vaccinia*, or cowpox, used by Jenner to protect against smallpox.

Grafting

Cells or organs from another individual usually survive natural resistance mechanisms but are attacked by the adaptive immune response, leading to **rejection**.

Autoimmunity

The body's own ('self') cells and molecules do not normally stimulate its adaptive immune responses because of a variety of special mechanisms which ensure a state of self-tolerance, but in certain circumstances they do stimulate a response and the body's own structures are attacked as if they were foreign, a condition called **autoimmunity** or **autoimmune disease**.

Hypersensitivity

Sometimes the result of specific memory is that re-exposure to the same stimulus, as well as or instead of eliminating the stimulus, has unpleasant or damaging effects on the body's own tissues. This is called **hypersensitivity**; examples are allergy (i.e. hay fever) and some forms of kidney disease. (Note, however, that the term 'allergy' is used by some immunologists to describe *all* alterations in responsiveness, in which case it also includes acquired resistance.)

Immunosuppression

Autoimmunity, hypersensitivity, and above all graft rejection, sometimes necessitate the suppression of adaptive immune responses by drugs or other means.

2 Natural and adaptive immune mechanisms

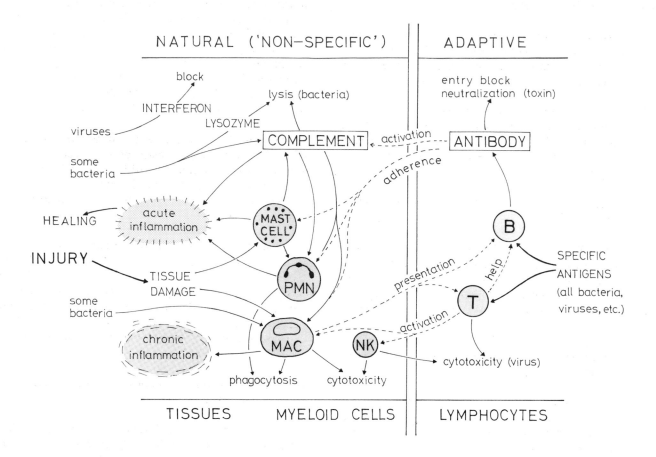

Just as resistance to disease can be natural (inborn) or acquired, the mechanisms mediating it can be correspondingly divided into **natural** (left) and **adaptive** (right), each composed of both **cellular** (lower) and **humoral** (i.e. free in serum or body fluids; upper half) elements. Adaptive mechanisms, more recently evolved, perform many of their functions by interacting with the older natural ones.

The mechanisms involved in natural immunity are largely the same as those responsible for non-specifically reacting to tissue damage, with the production of **inflammation** (cover up the right-hand part of the figure to appreciate this). However, some cells (e.g. macrophages) and some humoral factors (complement, lysozyme) do also have a limited ability to recognize and dispose of bacteria, while most cells can secrete interferon, which acts against viruses but not other types of organism. Thus the term 'non-specific', though often used as a synonym for 'natural', is not completely accurate.

Adaptive immunity is based on the special properties of **lymphocytes** (T and B, lower right), which can respond selectively to thousands of different non-self materials, or **'antigens'**, leading to specific memory and a permanently altered pattern of response—an *adaptation* to the animal's own surroundings. Adaptive mechanisms can function on their own against certain antigens (cover up the left-hand part of the figure), but the majority of their effects are exerted by means of the interaction of antibody with complement and the phagocytic cells of natural immunity, and of T cells with macrophages (broken lines). Through their activation of these natural mechanisms, adaptive responses frequently provoke **inflammation**, either acute or chronic; when it becomes a nuisance this is called **hypersensitivity**.

The individual elements of this highly simplified scheme are illustrated in more detail in the remainder of this book.

NATURAL IMMUNITY

Interferon A family of proteins produced rapidly by many cells in response to virus infection, which block the replication of virus in other cells.

Lysozyme (muramidase) An enzyme secreted by macrophages, which attacks the cell wall of some bacteria. Interferon and lysozyme are sometimes described as 'natural antibiotics'.

Complement A series of enzymes present in serum which when activated produce widespread inflammatory effects, as well as lysis of bacteria, etc. Some bacteria activate complement directly, while others only do so with the help of antibody (see Fig. 5).

Lysis Irreversible leakage of cell contents following membrane damage.

Mast cell A large tissue cell which releases inflammatory mediators when damaged, and also under the influence of antibody. By increasing vascular permeability, inflammation allows complement and cells to enter the tissues from the blood (see Fig. 6 for further details of this process).

PMN polymorphonuclear leucocyte, a short-lived 'scavenger' blood cell, whose granules contain powerful bactericidal enzymes.

MAC macrophage, a large tissue cell responsible for removing damaged tissue, cells, bacteria, etc. Both PMNs and macrophages come from the bone marrow, and are therefore known as **myeloid** cells.

Phagocytosis ('cell eating') Engulfment of a particle by a cell. Macrophages and PMNs (which used to be called 'microphages') are the most important phagocytic cells. The great majority of foreign materials entering the tissues are ultimately disposed of by this mechanism.

Cytotoxicity Macrophages can kill some targets (perhaps including tumour cells) without phagocytosing them, and there are a variety of other cells with cytoxic abilities.

NK (natural killer) cell A lymphocyte-like cell capable of killing some targets, notably virus-infected cells, but without the receptor or the fine specificity characteristic of true lymphocytes.

ADAPTIVE IMMUNITY

Antigen Strictly speaking, a substance which stimulates the production of **antibody**. The term is often applied, however, to substances that stimulate any type of adaptive immune response. Typically, antigens are foreign ('non-self') and either particulate (e.g. cells, bacteria, etc.) or large protein or polysaccharide molecules. But under special conditions small molecules and even 'self' components can become antigenic. The principal requirement of an antigen is some surface feature detectably foreign to the animal, though there is more to it than this (see Figs 17, 18).

Specific; specificity Terms used to denote the production of an immune response more or less selective for the stimulus, e.g. a lymphocyte which responds to, or an antibody which 'fits', a particular antigen. For example, antibody against measles virus will not bind to mumps virus: it is 'specific' for measles.

Lymphocyte A small cell found in blood, from which it recirculates through the tissues and back via the lymph, 'policing' the body for non-self material. Its ability to recognize individual antigens through its specialized surface receptors and to divide into numerous cells of identical specificity and long life-span, makes it the ideal cell for adaptive responses. Two major populations of lymphocytes are recognized: T and B.

B lymphocytes secrete antibody, the humoral element of adaptive immunity.

T ('thymus-derived') lymphocytes are further divided into subpopulations which 'help' B lymphocytes, kill virus-infected cells, activate macrophages, etc.

Antibody Serum globulins with a wide range of specificity for different antigens. Antibodies can bind to and neutralize bacterial toxins, and also, by binding to the surface of bacteria, viruses, or other parasites, increase their adherence to, and phagocytosis by, myeloid cells. This can be even further increased by the ability of many antibodies to activate complement.

Presentation of antigens to T and B cells by special macrophages is necessary for most adaptive responses; this is an example of 'reverse interaction' between adaptive and natural immune mechanisms.

Help by T cells is required for the secretion of most antibodies by B cells. There are also 'suppressor' T cells which have the opposite effect.

3 Evolution of immune mechanisms

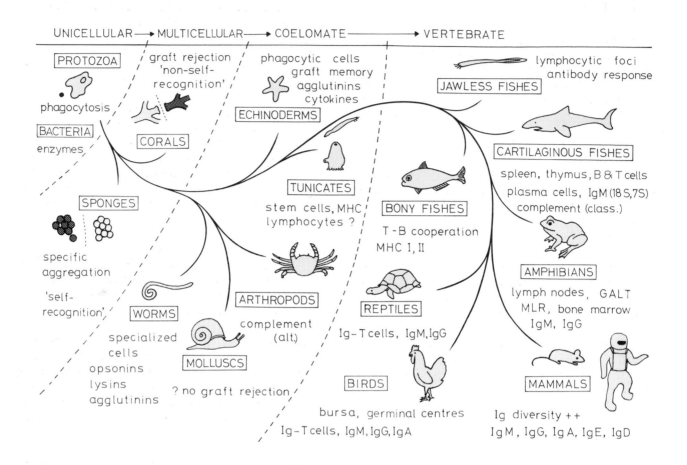

UNICELLULAR → MULTICELLULAR → COELOMATE → VERTEBRATE

PROTOZOA

phagocytosis

BACTERIA
enzymes

graft rejection
'non-self-
recognition'

CORALS

SPONGES

specific
aggregation

'self-
recognition'

WORMS

specialized
cells
opsonins
lysins
agglutinins

MOLLUSCS

? no graft rejection

phagocytic cells
graft memory
agglutinins
cytokines

ECHINODERMS

TUNICATES

stem cells, MHC
lymphocytes ?

ARTHROPODS

complement
(alt.)

JAWLESS FISHES

lymphocytic foci
antibody response

CARTILAGINOUS FISHES

spleen, thymus, B & T cells
plasma cells, IgM (18 S,7S)
complement (class.)

BONY FISHES

T - B cooperation
MHC I, II

REPTILES

Ig - T cells, IgM, IgG

BIRDS

bursa, germinal centres
Ig - T cells, IgM, IgG, IgA

AMPHIBIANS

lymph nodes, GALT
MLR, bone marrow
IgM, IgG

MAMMALS

Ig diversity + +
IgM, IgG, IgA, IgE, IgD

From the humble amoeba searching for food (top left) to the mammal with its sophisticated humoral and cellular immune mechanisms (bottom right), the process of **'self versus non-self recognition'** shows a steady development, keeping pace with the increasing need of animals to maintain their integrity in a hostile environment. The decision at which point 'immunity' appeared is thus a purely semantic one.

In this figure some of the important landmarks in this development are shown. Since most advances, once achieved, persist in subsequent species, they have for clarity been shown only where they are first thought to have appeared. It must be remembered that our knowledge of primitive animals is based largely on study of their modern descendants, all of whom evidently have immune systems adequate to their circumstances.

In so far as the T cell system is based on the cellular recognition of 'altered-self' or 'not-quite-self', it appears to have its roots considerably further back in evolution than antibody, which is roughly restricted to vertebrates. In mammals we can distinguish three separate **recognition systems**, based on molecules expressed on B cells only (antibody), on T cells only (the T cell receptor), and on a range of cells (the major histocompatibility complex, MHC), all of which look as if their genes evolved from a single primitive precursor (see Fig. 12 for further details). In addition there may be another set of 'receptors' on phagocytic cells (see Fig. 8), but neither the molecules nor the genes concerned have been identified yet.

Protozoa Lacking chlorophyll, these little animals must eat. Little is known about how they recognize 'food', but their surface proteins are under quite complex genetic control.

Bacteria We think of bacteria as parasites, but they themselves can suffer from infection by specialized viruses called bacteriophages. It is thought that the restriction endonucleases, so indispensable to the modern genetic engineer, have as their real function the recognition and destruction of viral DNA without damage to that of the host bacterium. Successful bacteriophages have evolved resistance to this, a beautiful example of natural immunity and its limitations.

Sponges Partly free-living, partly colonial, sponge cells use species-specific glycoproteins to identify 'self' and prevent hybrid colony formation. If forced together, non-identical colonies undergo necrosis at the contact zone, with accelerated breakdown of a second graft.

Corals Corals accept genetically identical grafts (syngrafts) but slowly reject non-identical ones (allografts) with damage to both partners. There is some evidence for specific memory of a previous rejection—i.e. of 'adaptive' immunity.

Worms A feature of all coelomate animals is cell specialization. In the earthworm coelom there are at least four cell types, some of which are involved in allograft rejection, while others may produce antibacterial factors; all are phagocytic.

Molluscs and **arthropods** are curious in apparently not showing graft rejection, but this may be due to the lack of heterogeneity in their MHC (see Fig. 13) rather than lack of a potential rejection system. However, humoral factors are prominent, possibly including the earliest complement (alternative pathway) components, which may be responsible for their resistance to some parasites.

Echinoderms The starfish is famous for Metchnikoff's classic demonstration of specialized phagocytic cells (1882). Allografts are rejected, with cellular infiltration, and there is a strong specific memory response. Molecules resembling the cytokines IL-1 (interleukin-1) and TNF (tumour necrosis factor) have been identified in these and other invertebrates.

Tunicates (e.g. *Amphioxus*, sea-squirts) These prevertebrates show several advanced features; self-renewing haemopoietic cells, lymphoid-like cells, and a single MHC controlling the rejection of foreign grafts.

Jawless fishes (cyclostomes, e.g. hagfish, lamprey) The earliest surviving vertebrates, with lymphoid cells organized into foci in the pharnyx and elsewhere, and the first definite antibody immunoglobulin (Ig), a labile four-chain molecule, produced specifically in response to a variety of antigens: a dramatic moment in the evolution of the immune system. Note that other molecules of the 'immunoglobulin superfamily', e.g. adhesion molecules, are already present in invertebrates such as the arthropods.

Cartilaginous fishes (e.g. sharks) The first appearance of the thymus, of the secondary antibody response, and of plasma cells (specialized for high-rate antibody secretion) marks another tremendous step. Ig chains are now disulphide-linked; the high and low molecular weight forms probably represent polymerization rather than class differences. Molecules of the classical complement pathway also make their appearance.

Bony fish The different responses to mitogens and the evidence for cell cooperation in antibody production suggest that T and B lymphocyte functions have begun to separate. Likewise, the MHC Class I and II antigens may have separated at this stage.

Amphibians The first appearance of another Ig class (IgG) and of the mixed-lymphocyte reaction (MLR). During morphogenesis (e.g. tadpole → frog) specific tolerance may develop towards the new antigens of the adult stage. Lymph nodes and gut-associated lymphoid tissue (GALT) and haemopoiesis in the bone marrow also appear for the first time.

Reptiles were previously thought to carry on their thymus cells Ig similar to that in serum, but the probability is that this is in fact the antecedent of the T cell receptor and that the antisera used for its detection 'cross-reacted' with Ig—a common problem in immunology.

Birds are unusual in producing their B lymphocytes exclusively in a special organ, the bursa of Fabricius, near the cloaca. Their complement system is also very different from that of mammals; for example Factor B appears to take the place of C4 and C2 (see Fig. 5).

Mammals are characterized more by Ig class and subclass diversity than by any further development of T cell functions. There are some curious variations; for example rats have unusually strong natural immunity and the Syrian hamster shows little or no graft rejection, but humans and mice are pretty similar to the immunologist.

4 Cells involved in immunity: the haemopoietic system

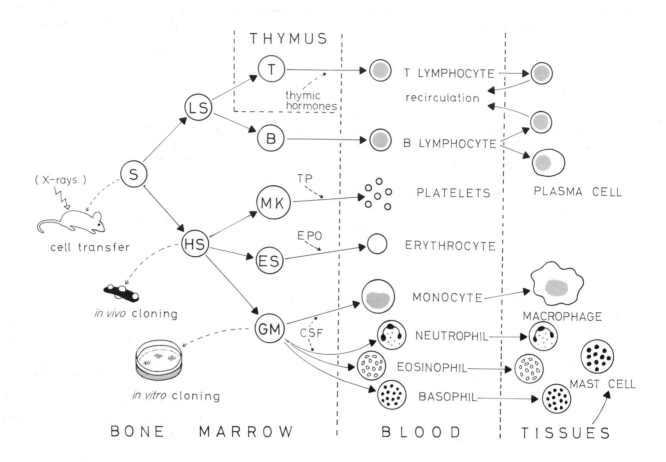

The great majority of cells involved in mammalian immunity are derived from precursors in the **bone marrow** (left half of figure) and circulate in the **blood**, entering and sometimes leaving the **tissues** when required.

The existence of the long-debated totipotent **stem cell** in the adult, retaining the 'embryonic' ability to differentiate into all types of blood cell, has been established by cell-transfer experiments and chromosome analysis in irradiated mice (centre left); stem cells are probably restricted to the bone marrow, and are very rare there (about one in 100 000 cells). By injecting small numbers of marrow cells, discrete spleen nodules, or 'in vivo clones' can be grown, whose morphology and differentiation can be studied in a more or less natural environment. Similar experiments in semi-solid culture conditions *in vitro* enable the clonal progeny of single marrow cells to be examined in complete isolation (lower left).

Unlike other haemopoietic cells, lymphocytes do not normally divide unless stimulated, and the propagation of lymphocyte clones usually requires repeated exposure to antigen and growth factors, followed by selection of specifically reactive cells. But T or B lymphocytes can be fused with a tumour cell, to produce an immortal hybrid clone or 'hybridoma', of great value in studying the properties of lymphocytes, which are complex and varied (see Fig. 9).

A note on terminology
Haematologists recognize many stages between stem cells and their fully differentiated progeny (e.g. for the red cells: proerythroblast; erythroblast, normoblast, erythrocyte). The suffix **blast** usually implies an early, dividing, relatively undifferentiated cell, but is also used to describe lymphocytes that have been stimulated, e.g. by antigen, and are about to divide; whence the term 'blast transformation'.

S Stem cell; the totipotent marrow cell, of proved existence but uncertain morphology.

LS Lymphoid stem cell, presumed to be capable of differentiating into T or B lymphocytes.

HS Haemopoietic stem cell; the precursor of spleen nodules and probably able to differentiate into all but the lymphoid pathways.

ES Erythroid stem cell, destined to differentiate into erythrocytes. Haematologists distinguish the BFU (burst-forming unit) and the later CFU (colony-forming unit) on the basis of their growth patterns *in vitro*.

EPO Erythropoietin; a glycoprotein hormone formed in the kidney in response to hypoxia, which accelerates the differentiation of erythrocyte precursors, and thus adjusts the production of red cells to the demand for their oxygen-carrying capacity—a typical example of 'negative feedback'.

GM Granulocyte–monocyte common precursor; a cell capable of differentiating into various cells of the myeloid series depending on the presence of growth- or 'colony-stimulating' factors.

Neutrophil (polymorph)   The commonest leucocyte of the blood, a short-lived phagocytic cell whose granules contain numerous bactericidal substances.

Eosinophil   A leucocyte whose large refractile granules contain a number of highly basic or 'cationic' proteins, possibly important in killing larger parasites including worms.

Basophil   A leucocyte whose large basophilic granules contain heparin and vasoactive amines, important in the inflammatory response.

The above three cell types are often collectively referred to as 'granulocytes.'

Monocyte   The largest nucleated cell of the blood, developing into a macrophage when it migrates into the tissues.

Macrophage   The principal resident phagocyte of the tissues and serous cavities such as the pleura and peritoneum.

CSF   Colony-stimulating factor(s); substances produced by various kinds of cell, required for the differentiation of granulocytes and monocytes. Some of the CSFs are now available in pure form, thanks to genetic engineering, and somewhat surprisingly each of them appears to have multiple effects so that no individual cell type is under the control of any single factor. As with the interferons and interleukins (see Fig. 22), CSFs seem to respond to overall requirements—a much more 'holistic' view of regulation than used to prevail.

MK   Megakaryocyte; the parent cell of the blood platelets.

TP   Thrombopoietin; a hormone which regulates the production of platelets.

T   Thymus-derived (or -processed) lymphocyte.

Thymic hormones   Numerous small peptides extracted from thymic epithelium (e.g. 'thymosin') are thought by some to assist the differentiation of T lymphocytes (see Figs 9–11 for further details of lymphocyte development).

B   Bone marrow- (or, in birds, bursa-) derived lymphocyte, the precursor of antibody-forming cells. In foetal life, the liver may play the role of 'bursa'.

Plasma cell   A B cell in its high-rate antibody-secreting state. Despite their name, plasma cells are seldom seen in the blood, but are found in spleen, lymph nodes, etc.; whenever antibody is being made.

Mast cell   A large tissue cell similar in appearance and function to the basophil, but thought not to originate from the bone marrow. Mast cells are easily triggered by tissue damage to initiate the inflammatory response. (See Fig. 32 for details of mast cell sub-populations.)

5 Complement

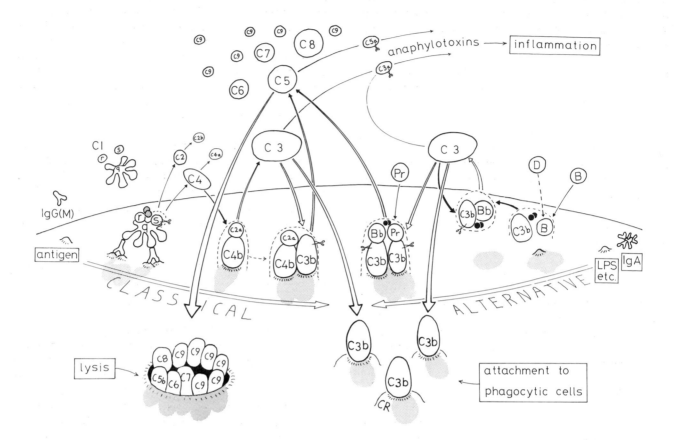

Fifteen or more serum components constitute the **complement** system, whose sequential activation and assembly into functional units leads to three main effects: release of peptides active in **inflammation** (top right), deposition of C3b, a powerful attachment-promoter (or 'opsonin') for **phagocytosis**, on cell membranes (bottom right), and membrane damage resulting in *lysis* (bottom left). Together these make it an important part of the defences against micro-organisms. Defects of some components can predispose to severe infections, particularly bacterial (see Fig. 38).

The upper half of the figure represents the serum, or 'fluid' phase, the lower half the cell surface, where activation (indicated by dotted haloes) and assembly largely occur. Activation of complement can proceed by two distinct routes, the '**classical**' (because first described) pathway, initiated by the binding of specific antibody of the IgG or IgM class (see Fig. 16) to surface antigens (centre left), and the '**alternative**', but probably more primitive, pathway, initiated by a variety of polysaccharides and by some antibodies (centre right). Some of the steps are dependent on the divalent ions Ca^{2+} (shaded circles) or Mg^{2+} (black circles).

Activation is usually limited to the immediate vicinity by the very short life of the active products, and in some cases there are special inactivators (✗). Nevertheless, excessive complement activation can cause unpleasant side-effects (see Fig. 33).

CLASSICAL PATHWAY

For many years this was the only way in which complement was known to be activated. The essential feature is the requirement for a specific antigen–antibody interaction, leading via components C1, C2 and C4 to the formation of a 'convertase' which splits C3.

Ig IgM and some subclasses of IgG (in the human, IgG3, 1 and 2), when bound to antigen are recognized by Clq to initiate the classical pathway.

C1 A Ca^{2+} dependent union of three components: Clq (MW 400 000), a curious protein with six valencies for Ig linked by collagen-like fibrils, which activates in turn Clr (MW 170 000) and Cls (MW 80 000), a serine esterase which goes on to attack C2 and C4.

C2 (MW 120 000), split by Cls into small (C2b) and large (C2a) fragments.

C4 (MW 240 000), likewise split into C4a (small) and C4b (large). C4b and C2a then join together and attach to the antigen–antibody complex, or to the membrane in the case of a cell-bound antigen, forming a 'C3 convertase'. Note that some complementologists prefer to reverse the names of C2a and b, so that for both C2 and C4 the 'a' peptide is the smaller one.

C3 (MW 180 000), the central component of all complement reactions, split by its convertase into a small (C3a) and a large fragment (C3b). Some of the C3b is deposited on the membrane, where it serves as an attachment site for phagocytic polymorphs and macrophages, which have receptors for it; some remains associated with C2a and C4b, forming a 'C5 convertase'. Two 'C3b inactivator' enzymes rapidly inactivate C3b, releasing the fragment C3c and leaving membrane-bound C3d.

C5 (MW 180 000), split by its convertase into C5a, a small peptide which, together with C3a (anaphylotoxins), acts on mast cells, polymorphs and smooth muscle to promote the inflammatory response, and C5b, which initiates the assembly of C6, 7, 8 and 9 into the membrane-damaging or 'lytic' unit.

CR Complement receptor. Three types of molecule that bind different products of C3 breakdown are found on cell surfaces: CR1 on red cells, CR1 and CR3 on phagocytic cells, where they act as opsonins (see Fig. 8) and CR2 on B lymphocytes where it may be involved in the induction of memory but is also, unfortunately, the receptor via which the Epstein–Barr virus gains entry (see Fig. 26).

ALTERNATIVE PATHWAY

6 Acute inflammation

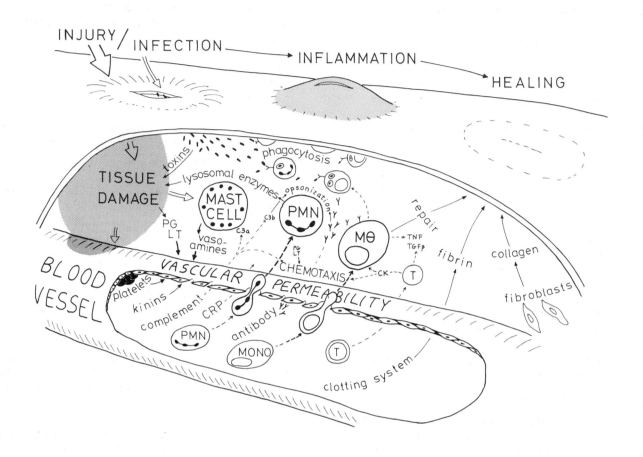

Whether **inflammation** should be considered part of immunology is a problem for the teaching profession, not for the body—which combats infection by all the means at its disposal, including mechanisms also involved in the response to and repair of other types of damage.

In this simplified scheme, which should be read from left to right, are shown the effects of **injury** to tissues (top left) and to blood vessels (bottom left). The small black rods represent bacterial **infection**, a very common cause of inflammation and of course a frequent accompaniment of injury. Note the central role of **permeability of the vascular endothelium** in allowing access of blood

cells and serum components (lower half) to the tissues (upper half), which also accounts for the main symptoms of inflammation—redness, warmth, swelling and pain.

It can be seen that the 'adaptive' (or 'immunological') functions of antibody and lymphocytes largely operate to amplify or focus pre-existing 'natural' mechanisms; quantitatively, however, they are so important that they frequently make the difference between life and death. Further details of the role of antibody and lymphocytes in inflammation can be found in Figs 31–34.

Mast cell A large tissue cell with basophilic granules containing vasoactive amines and heparin. It degranulates readily in response to injury by trauma, heat, UV light, etc. and also in some allergic conditions (see Fig. 32).

PG, LT Prostaglandins and leukotrienes; a family of unsaturated fatty acids (MW 300–400) derived by metabolism of arachidonic acid, a component of most cell membranes. Individual PGs and LTs have different but overlapping effects; together they are responsible for the induction of pain, fever, vascular permeability and chemotaxis of PMN, and some of them also inhibit lymphocyte functions.

Vasoamines Vasoactive amines; e.g. histamine, 5-hydroxytryptamine, produced by mast cells, basophils and platelets, and causing increased capillary permeability.

Complement A cascading sequence of serum proteins, activated either directly ('alternate pathway') or via antigen–antibody interaction (see Fig. 5 for details of the individual components).

C3a and **C5a** which stimulate release by mast cells of their vasoactive amines, are known as anaphylotoxins.

Opsonization C3b attached to a particle promotes sticking to phagocytic cells because of their 'C3 receptors'. Antibody, if present, augments this by binding to 'Fc receptors'.

CRP C-reactive protein (MW 130 000), a pentameric globulin which appears in the serum within hours of tissue damage or infection, and whose ancestry goes back to the invertebrates. It binds to phosphorylcholine, which is found on the surface of many bacteria, fixes complement and promotes phagocytosis, thus it may play an antibody-like role in some bacterial infections. Proteins whose serum concentration increases during inflammation are called **'acute phase proteins'**; they include CRP and many complement components, as well as other microbe-binding molecules and enzyme inhibitors. This **acute phase response** can be viewed as a rapid, not very specific, attempt to deal with more or less any type of infection or damage.

Kinin system A series of serum peptides sequentially activated to cause vasodilation and increased permeability.

PMN Polymorphonuclear leucocyte; the major mobile phagocytic cell, whose prompt arrival in the tissues plays a vital part in removing invading bacteria.

Mono Monocyte; the precursor of tissue macrophages (Mθ in the figure) which is responsible for removing damaged tissue as well as micro-organisms.

Lysosomal enzymes Bactericidal enzymes released from the lysosomes of PMNs, monocytes and macrophages, e.g. lysozyme, myeloperoxidase.

Chemotaxis C5a, C3a, leukotrienes and some lymphocyte products stimulate PMNs and monocytes to move into the tissues. Movement towards the site of inflammation is called chemotaxis, and is presumably due to the cells' ability to detect a concentration gradient of chemotactic factors; random increases of movement are called chemokinesis.

T T lymphocyte, undergoing **blast** transformation if stimulated by antigen, as in the case of most infections.

CK Cytokines; lymphocyte and macrophage products affecting both cell types as well as other tissue cells. Two of them, TNF (tumour necrosis factor) and TGFβ (transforming growth factor), are involved in healing and repair (see Fig. 22 for details).

Clotting system Intimately bound up with complement and kinins because of several shared activation steps. Blood clotting is a vital part of the healing process.

Fibrin the end product of blood clotting and, in the tissues, the matrix into which fibroblasts migrate to initiate healing.

Fibroblast an important tissue cell which migrates into the fibrin clot and secretes **collagen**, an enormously strong polymerizing molecule giving the healing wound its strength and elasticity. Subsequently new blood capillaries sprout into the area, leading eventually to the restoration of the normal architecture.

7 Phagocytic cells: the reticulo-endothelial system

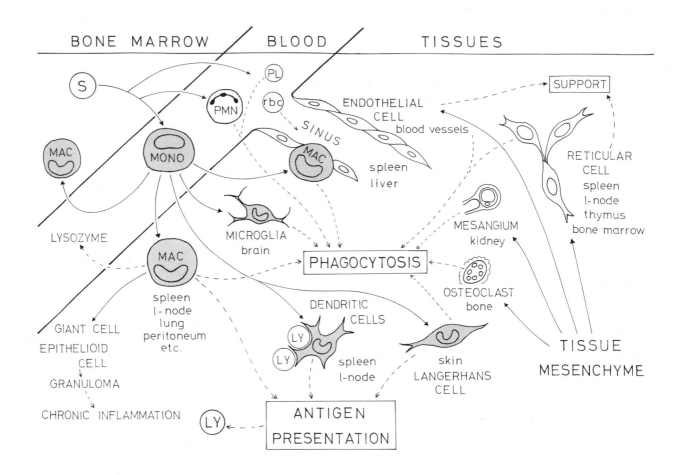

Particulate matter which finds its way into the blood or tissues is rapidly removed by cells, and the property of taking up dyes, colloids, etc., was used by anatomists to define a body-wide system of phagocytic cells known as the **'reticulo-endothelial system'** (RES), consisting of the vascular endothelium and reticular tissue cells (top right), and —supposedly descended from these—various types of macrophages whose routine functions included clearing up the body's own debris and killing and digesting bacteria.

However, more modern work has shown a fundamental distinction between those phagocytic cells derived from the bone marrow via the blood monocyte (shaded) and others formed locally from the tissues themselves (right side of figure). Ironically, neither reticular nor endothelial cells are outstandingly phagocytic, their function being mainly structural.

More recently still, attention has focused on the interactions between the RES and adaptive immunity. The role of antibody in amplifying phagocytosis and of T lymphocytes in activating other macrophage functions is discussed in Figs 8 and 34, but it is worth noting here that neither B nor T lymphocytes can normally respond to foreign antigens unless the latter are properly **'presented'**. It used to be assumed that the presenting cells were typical macrophages, but it is now clear that there are special separate populations of cells in the skin and the lymphoid organs (lower centre) with the ability to bind protein antigens, break them down into small peptides, which associate with MHC molecules and are then recognized by T cells (see Figs 14, 19). When this process is fully understood, there may be some hope of a rational classification of this whole group of cells.

Endothelial cell The inner lining of blood vessels, able to take up dyes, etc., but not truly phagocytic. There is, however, evidence that endothelial cells can present antigen to lymphocytes under some circumstances, and they can both produce and respond to cytokines rather as macrophages do.

Reticular cell The main supporting or 'stromal' cell of lymphoid organs, usually associated with the collagen-like reticulin fibres, and not easily distinguished from fibroblasts or from other branching or 'dendritic' cells (see below)—whence a great deal of confusion.

Mesangium Mesangial cells give support to the glomerulus, and may phagocytose material deposited in it, particularly complexes of antigen and antibody.

Osteoclast A large multinucleate cell responsible for resorbing and so shaping bone. There is some evidence that its function can be regulated by T lymphocytes.

Dendritic cells The weakly phagocytic **Langerhans cell** of the epidermis, and somewhat similar but non-phagocytic cells in the lymphoid follicles of the spleen and lymph nodes, are the main agents of T cell stimulation; T cells recognize foreign antigens in association with cell-surface antigens coded for by the MHC, a genetic region intimately involved in immune responses of all kinds (see Figs 13, 14, 19). There are separate follicular dendritic cells for presenting antigen to B cells. All cells of this type appear to be derived ultimately from the bone marrow.

Ly Lymphocytes are often found in close contact with dendritic cells; this is presumably where antigen presentation and T–B cell cooperation take place (see Fig. 17).

S The totipotent bone marrow stem cell, giving rise to all the cells found in blood.

PL Blood platelets, though primarily involved in clotting, are able to phagocytose antigen–antibody complexes.

RBC Antigen–antibody complexes which have bound complement can become attached to red blood cells via the CR1 receptor (see Fig. 5) on the latter, which then transport the complexes to the liver for removal by macrophages. This is sometimes referred to as 'immune adherence'.

PMN Polymorphonuclear leucocyte, the major phagocytic cell of the blood; not, however, conventionally considered as part of the RES.

Mono Monocyte, formed in the marrow and travelling via the blood to the tissues, where it matures into a macrophage. It is likely, though not proved, that the specialized antigen-presenting cells also develop from monocytes.

Mac Macrophage, the resident and long-lived tissue phagocyte. Macrophages may be either free in the tissues, or 'fixed' in the walls of blood sinuses, where they monitor the blood for particles, effete red cells, etc. This activity is strongest in the liver, where the macrophages are called Kupffer cells. Macrophages (and polymorphs) have the valuable ability to recognize not only foreign matter but also antibody and/or complement bound to it, which greatly enhances phagocytosis (see Fig. 8).

Sinus Tortuous channels in liver, spleen, etc., through which blood passes to reach the veins, allowing the lining macrophages to remove damaged or antibody-coated cells and other particles. This process is so effective that a large injection of, for example, carbon particles, can be removed from the blood within minutes, leaving the liver and spleen visibly black.

Microglia The phagocytic cells of the brain, thought to be derived from incoming blood monocytes.

Lysozyme An important anti-bacterial enzyme secreted into the blood by macrophages. Macrophages also produce other 'natural' humoral factors such as interferon and many complement components, cytotoxic factors, etc.

Giant cell; epithelioid cell Macrophage-derived cells typically found at sites of chronic inflammation; by coalescing into a solid mass, or **granuloma**, they localize and wall off irritant or indigestible materials (see Fig. 34).

8 Phagocytosis

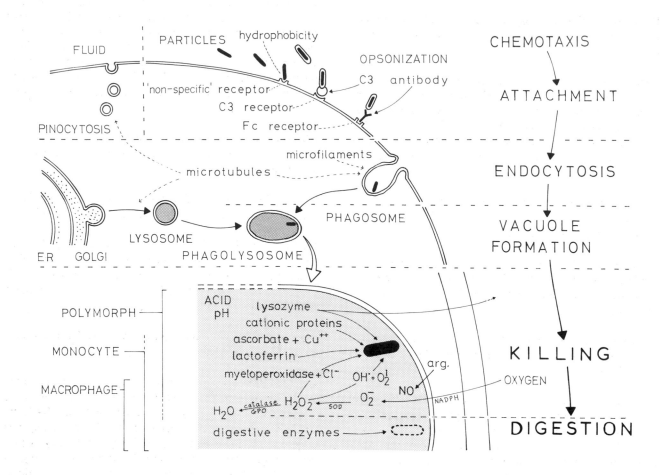

Numerous cells are able to ingest foreign materials, but the ability to increase this activity in response to opsonization by antibody and/or complement, so as to acquire antigen-specificity, is restricted to cells of the myeloid series, principally the **polymorphs**, **monocytes**, and **macrophages**; these are sometimes termed 'professional' phagocytes.

Apart from some variations in their content of lysosomal enzymes, all myeloid cells use essentially similar mechanisms to phagocytose foreign objects, consisting of a sequence of **attachment** (top), endocytosis or **ingestion** (centre), and **digestion** (bottom). In the figure this process is shown for a typical bacterium (small black rods). In general, bacteria with **capsules** (shown outlined) are not phagocytosed unless opsonized, whereas many non-capsulated ones do not require this. There are certain differences

between phagocytic cells; for example polymorphs are very short-lived (hours or days) and often die in the process of phagocytosis, while macrophages, which lack some of the more destructive enzymes, usually survive to phagocytose again. Also, macrophages can actively secrete some of their enzymes, e.g. lysozyme. There are surprisingly large species differences in the proportions of the various lysosomal enzymes.

Several of the steps in phagocytosis shown in the figure may be specifically defective for genetic reasons (see Fig. 38), as well as being actively inhibited by particular micro-organisms (see Figs 25, 27, 29). In either case the result is a failure to eliminate micro-organisms or foreign material properly, leading to chronic infection and/or chronic inflammation.

Chemotaxis The process by which cells are attracted towards bacteria, etc., often by following a gradient of molecules released by the microbe.

Pinocytosis 'Cell drinking'; the ingestion of soluble materials, conventionally applied to particles under 1 μm in diameter.

Hydrophobicity Hydrophobic groups tend to attach to the hydrophobic surface of cells; this may explain the 'recognition' of damaged cells, denatured proteins, etc. Bacterial capsules, largely polysaccharide, reduce hydrophobicity and block attachment, an important escape mechanism used by many of the most virulent bacteria (see Fig. 25).

Non-specific receptor Another view is that phagocytic cells have surface structures complementary to the wide range of materials they recognize and attach to.

C3 receptor Phagocytic cells (and some lymphocytes) can bind C3b, produced from C3 by activation by bacteria, etc., either directly or via antibody (see Fig. 5 for details of the receptors).

Fc receptor Phagocytic cells (and most lymphocytes, platelets, etc.) can bind the Fc portion of antibody, especially of the IgG class.

Opsonization refers to the promotion or enhancement of attachment via the C3 or Fc receptor. Discovered by Almroth Wright and made famous by G.B. Shaw in 'The Doctor's Dilemma', opsonization is probably the single most important process by which antibody helps to overcome infections, particularly bacterial.

Phagosome A vacuole formed by the internalization of surface membrane along with an attached particle.

Microtubules Short rigid structures composed of the protein tubulin which arrange themselves into channels for vacuoles, etc. to travel within the cell, and also serve to stiffen the membrane.

Microfilaments Contractile protein (actin) filaments responsible for membrane activities such as pinocytosis and phagosome formation. There are also intermediate filaments composed of the protein vimentin.

ER Endoplasmic reticulum; a membranous system of sacs and tubules with which ribosomes are associated in the synthesis of many proteins for secretion.

Golgi The region where products of the ER are packaged into vesicles.

Lysosome A membrane-bound package of hydrolytic enzymes usually active at acid pH (e.g. acid phosphatase, DNAase). Lysosomes are found in almost all cells, and are vehicles for secretion as well as digestion. They are prominent in macrophages and polymorphs, which also have separate vesicles containing lysozyme and other enzymes; together with lysosomes these constitute the **granules** whose staining patterns characterize the various types of polymorph (neutrophil, basophil, eosinophil). Newly formed lysosomes not containing any substrate are sometimes called 'primary'.

Phagolysosome A vacuole formed by the fusion of a phagosome and lysosome(s), in which micro-organisms are killed and digested.

Lactoferrin A protein that inhibits bacteria by depriving them of iron, which it binds with an extremely high affinity.

Cationic proteins Examples are 'phagocytin', 'leukin'; microbicidal agents found in some polymorph granules. Eosinophils are particularly rich in cationic proteins, which can be secreted when the cell 'degranulates', making them highly cytotoxic cells.

Ascorbate interacts with copper ions and hydrogen peroxide, and can be bactericidal.

Oxygen Intracellular killing of many bacteria requires the uptake of oxygen by the phagocytic cell, i.e. it is 'aerobic'. Through a series of enzyme reactions including NADPH oxidase and superoxide dismutase (SOD) this oxygen is progressively reduced to superoxide (O_2^-), hydrogen peroxide (H_2O_2) and hydroxyl ions (**OH**) and singlet oxygen (O_2^1). These 'free radicals' are highly toxic to many micro-organisms but they act only briefly because of cellular enzymes such as **catalase** and glutathione peroxidase (**GPO**) which remove them. Not surprisingly, some bacteria make such enzymes too (see Fig. 23). Nitric oxide (**NO**) produced from arginine has recently been also shown to be toxic.

Myeloperoxidase An important microbicidal enzyme in conjunction with hydrogen peroxide and halide (e.g. chloride) ions. It is absent from mature macrophages but may be partly replaced by catalase.

Lysozyme (muramidase) lyses many saprophytes (e.g. *Micrococcus lysodeicticus*) and some pathogenic bacteria damaged by antibody and/or complement. It is a major secretory product of macrophages, present in the blood at levels of micrograms per ml.

Digestive enzymes The enzymes by which lysosomes are usually identified, such as acid phosphatase, lipase, elastase, β glucuronidase, and the cathepsins thought to be important in antigen processing.

9 Lymphocytes

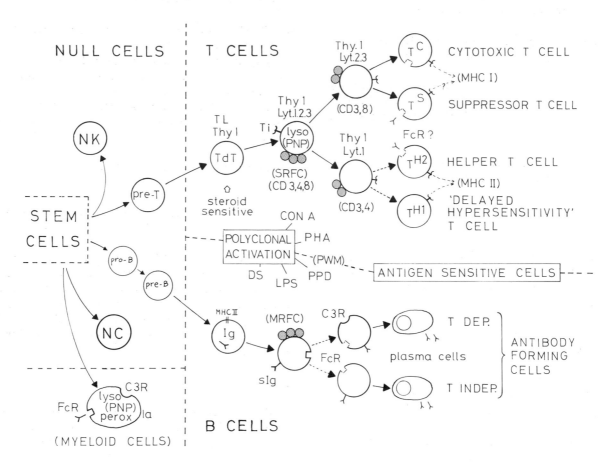

As befits the cell of adaptive immunity, the lymphocyte has several unique features: restricted receptors permitting each cell to respond to an individual antigen (the basis of **specificity**), clonal proliferation and long life span (the basis of **memory**), and recirculation from the tissues back into the bloodstream, which ensures that specific memory following a local response has a bodywide **distribution**.

The discovery in the early 1960s of the two major lymphocyte subpopulations, **T** (thymus-dependent; top) and **B** (bursa or bone marrow-dependent; bottom), had roughly the same impact on cellular immunology as the double helix on molecular biology. The first property of T cells to be distinguished was that of 'helping' B cells to make antibody, but further subdivisions have subsequently come to light, based on both functional and physical differences; four types of T cell are now recognized (top right). In the figure, the main surface features (or 'markers') of the various stages of lymphocyte differentiation are given for the mouse, with some special markers of human sub-populations shown in brackets or inside the cell. The latter have been of particular value in classifying lymphoid and myeloid malignancies (leukaemia).

Cells resembling lymphocytes, but without characteristic T or B cell markers are referred to as 'null' (left). This group probably includes early T cells, B cells and monocytes, as well as the 'natural killer' cells possibly important in tumour and virus immunity. In blood and lymphoid organs, up to 10% of lymphocytes are 'null'.

In one of the most exciting recent developments in biology, it has been found possible to perpetuate individual lymphocytes by fusing them with a tumour cell. In the case of B lymphocytes, this can mean an endless supply of individual, or **monoclonal**, antibodies, with far-reaching applications in the diagnosis and treatment of disease and the study of cell surfaces. Indeed, the classification of lymphocytes themselves, and of most other cells too, is now mainly based on patterns of reactivity with a large range of monoclonal typing antisera (see Appendix 3, Section 43).

In the case of T cells, it is also possible to keep them proliferating indefinitely in culture by judicious application of their specific antigen and non-specific growth factors such as IL-2 (see Fig. 22). The properties of the resulting **lines** or **clones** should eventually help in the understanding of normal T cell function, but so far they seem to have generated mainly confusion.

NULL CELLS

NK Natural killer cell, cytotoxic to some tumours, apparently in the absence of antibody. Some NK cells may belong to the T cell lineage but lack T cell receptors.

NC Natural cytotoxic cells, similar to NK cells but probably more closely related to macrophages than T cells.

Myeloid cells Monocytes, macrophages and granulocytes are effective in antibody-dependent cytotoxicity (ADCC), as are some T and NK cells. Collectively, these are referred to as K cells.

FcR 'Fc receptor'; a receptor for the Fc portion of antibody, especially IgG, which links the ADCC effector cell to its target.

T CELLS

TdT Terminal deoxynucleotidyl transferase, a DNA polymerase found mainly in cortical, and therefore young, thymocytes, probably involved in rearrangement of the genes for the T cell receptor.

Ti The T cell receptor for antigen, analogous to surface Ig on the B cell (see Fig. 14).

PNP Purine nucleoside phosphorylase, a purine salvage enzyme, found in human T cells and monocytes, but not B cells; a potentially useful marker.

Lyso Lysosomal enzymes (e.g. acid phosphatase, esterases, etc.) are found in myeloid cells and to a lesser extent in T cells.

TL Originally 'thymus leukaemia'; a surface antigen of leukaemic and normal mouse thymocytes, absent from mature T cells.

Thy 1 Originally 'theta'; a mouse T cell surface antigen existing in two allelic forms. It is also found on some brain and skin cells.

CD, LyT Based on reactivity with various monoclonal antibodies recognizing surface molecules, T and B cells can be classified and their lineages worked out. A full list of CD numbers is given in Appendix 3 (Section 43), but it should be noted that the older functional names (C3 receptor, sheep-cell receptor, etc.) are still in use, and so are the LyT numbers for mouse cells.

Polyclonal activation Stimulation of a substantial number of lymphocytes, i.e. many clones, rather than the few or single clones normally stimulated by an antigen. Since the first sign of activation is often mitosis, polyclonal activators are sometimes known as 'mitogens'. A surprising number of such 'lectins' are of plant origin, e.g. concanavalin A (CON

A) and phytohaemagglutinin (PHA), and act by a complementary interaction with surface carbohydrates on the cell; this is probably quite fortuitous and has no significance except as a most useful 'marker'.

SRFC Sheep rosette-forming cell; most human T cells bind sheep RBC to make 'rosettes' *in vitro*. The T cells of many species react in the same way with selected heterologous erythrocytes (e.g. cat: guinea-pig). Like the response to mitogens, this is a useful marker without functional significance—which needs to be distinguished from the use of sheep red cells as *antigens*, very common in experimental immunology.

Cytotoxic T cell A key cell in virus immunity (see Figs 19, 26).

Suppressor T cell Related, and possibly identical to, the above. It can inhibit both B and T cell responses.

Helper T cell The CD4 T cell essential for most antibody and cell-mediated responses (see Figs 17, 19). There is a suggestion that different CD4 T cells make the different sets of cytokines needed for antibody and cell-mediated immunity (CMI); these are sometimes called TH2 and TH1 respectively, the latter being also known as **delayed hypersensitivity** T cells.

B CELLS

Ig; sIg Immunoglobulin, at first cytoplasmic and later surface bound, is the key feature of B cells, through which they recognize specific antigens (see Figs 12, 14).

MHC II Antigens coded by the Class II region of the major histocompatibility complex, expressed mainly on B cells and macrophages, and involved in the interaction of these with the CD4 type of T cells (see Figs 15, 17).

CR2 Receptors for C3 on B cells may be involved in the generation of memory responses.

DS Dextran sulphate. **LPS** lipopolysaccharide, e.g. *Salmonella* endotoxin. **PPD** purified protein derivative (or tuberculin). The above are normally mitogenic only for B cells, possibly at different stages.

PWM Pokeweed mitogen, mitogenic for both T and B cells when both are present. There is unfortunately no ideal mitogen for human B cells.

MRFC Mouse rosette-forming cell; mature human B cells and B cell leukaemias bind mouse erythrocytes *in vitro*.

T dep., T indep. Some antibody formation, especially IgM, does not require T cell help, and is called 'thymus independent'. It involves different B cells and may be evolutionarily more primitive.

10 Primary lymphoid organs and lymphopoiesis

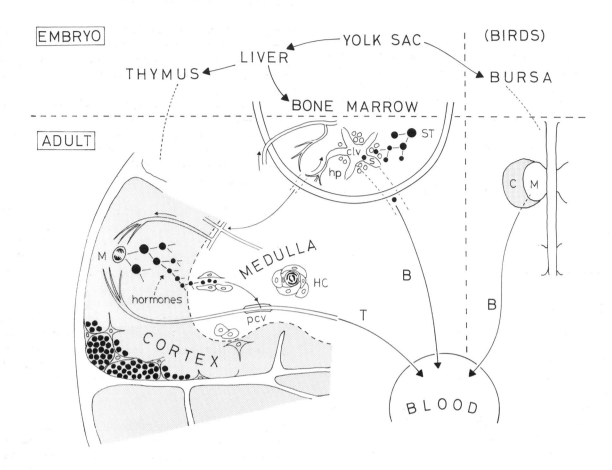

The first strong evidence for distinct lymphocyte populations was the complementary effects in birds of early removal of the **thymus** (which mainly affects cell-mediated immunity) and the **bursa of Fabricius** (which affects antibody responses). A continuing puzzle has been the identification of what represents the bursa in mammals; despite a phase when 'gut-associated lymphoid tissue' was a popular candidate, current opinion considers there to be no true analogue, the liver taking over the function of B cell maturation in the foetus, the bone marrow in the adult.

Another vexed question is why so many cells die in the thymus—up to 90% according to some calculations—and an attractive idea, which has recently received considerable support, is that it is here that self-reactive cells are weeded out. If the mysterious Hassal's corpuscles turn out to be the site of this process, two enigmas will be resolved at once.

Nor are these the only controversies involving the thymus. The status of its presumed hormones, such as 'thymosin', is still hotly disputed; there are conflicting ideas as to whether all T cells pass from the medulla to the cortex before leaving, or whether a distinct subpopulation leaves directly from the cortex; it is still not totally clear what role the thymus plays in determining the pattern of T cell reactivity to antigens, and finally, despite the lack of solid evidence, many people feel the thymus has something to do with cancer and ageing. (One wonders how long it will be before someone revives Galen's theory that it is the site of the soul!)

YOLK SAC

The source of the earliest haemopoietic tissue, including the lymphocyte precursors.

BURSA

In birds, B lymphocytes differentiate in the bursa of Fabricius, a cloacal outgrowth with many crypts and follicles, which reaches its maximum size a few weeks after birth and thereafter atrophies. Despite claims for the appendix, tonsil, etc., there is probably no mammalian analogue.

M Medulla; the region where the first stem cells colonize the bursal follicles.

C Cortex; the site of proliferation of the B lymphocytes.

LIVER

During foetal life in mammals, the major haemopoietic and lymphopoietic organ.

BONE MARROW

ST Stem cells for the B cell series.

HP Haemopoietic area. The anatomical location of lymphopoiesis in liver and bone marrow is not exactly known, but it presumably proceeds alongside the other haemopoietic pathways, in close association with macrophages and reticular cells. At least 70% of B cells die before release, probably because of faulty rearrangement of their immunoglobulin genes (see Fig. 15) or excessive self-reactivity.

S Sinus, collecting differentiated cells

CLV Central longitudinal vein, collecting cells from the sinuses for discharge into the blood.

THYMUS

Like the bursa, the thymus reaches its largest size in early life, though the subsequent atrophy is slower. In the mouse it contains almost exclusively cells of the T series, but in some animals there may be variable numbers of B cells as well. T cell precursors are derived, via the blood, from the bone marrow; they may undergo some degree of differentiation in the marrow under the influence of thymic hormones, but most of their maturation occurs within the thymus itself. There is evidence that at some stage they develop within specialized epithelial 'nurse' cells.

Recent work on the specificity of T cells (see Figs 17, 19) and the key role of the MHC (see also Fig. 13), has suggested that T cells learn first to recognize 'self' antigens, and that this occurs in the thymus (see below).

Hormones Numerous soluble factors extracted from the thymus have been shown to stimulate the maturation of T cells, as judged by function or surface markers or both. There is no agreed terminology, and the following list is far from complete:

Thymosin α1 (MW 3108), β1 (MW 8451), β4 (MW 4982)
Thymopoietin I, II (MW 9562)
Thymosin (MW 3108), B, (MW 8451), B4 (MW 4982)
Thymic humoral factor (MW 3220)
Thymostimulin (MW 12 000)
Facteur thymique serique (MW 857).

Cortex Dark-staining outer part packed with lymphocytes, compartmentalized by elongated epithelial cells. It may be here that newly entered cells from the bone marrow acquire 'MHC restriction' (see Fig. 13), and in the process become committed to the expression of either CD4 or CD8.

M Mitotic figures are common; it is thought that about eight divisions occur between the precursor cell and the exported T cell. Pyknotic nuclei are also common, suggesting that many cells die without leaving the thymus, by a carefully programmed process known as apoptosis, followed by phagocytosis by macrophages.

Medulla Inner, predominantly epithelial part, to which some (perhaps all) cortical lymphocytes migrate before export. Here the developing T cells are thought to encounter special antigen-presenting ('dendritic') cells and acquire 'self-tolerance' (see Fig. 20). How any T cells survive the ordeal of positive followed by negative selection, both of which seem to be directed by MHC molecules, is still a bit of a mystery. It is also not known what dictates whether a T cell will express the αβ or γδ receptor (see Fig. 14).

PCV Post-capillary venule, through which lymphocytes enter the thymic veins and ultimately the blood.

HC Hassal's corpuscle—a structure peculiar to the thymus, in which epithelial cells become concentrically compressed and keratinized. It is suspected by some of being the site of production of thymic hormones.

11 Secondary lymphoid organs and lymphocyte traffic

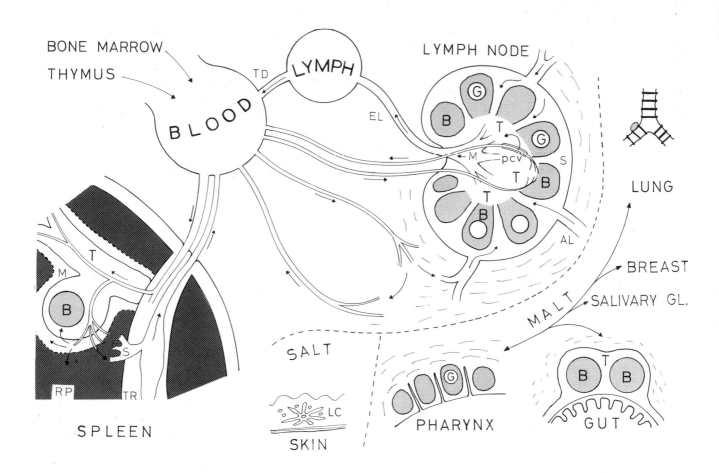

The ability to **recirculate** from blood to tissues and back through the lymphoid system is unique to lymphocytes and, coupled with their long life span and specificity for individual antigens, equips them for their central role in adaptive immune responses.

The thorough mixing of lymphocytes, particularly in the **spleen** and **lymph nodes**, ensures the maximum contact of antigen-presenting cells that have newly encountered antigen, with T and B lymphocytes potentially able to respond, which would otherwise be a very rare event. The bodywide dissemination of expanded T and B populations in readiness for a second encounter with the same antigen ensures that 'memory' is available at all sites.

There is a tendency for different types of lymphocyte to 'home' to different regions in the lymphoid organs (**T** and **B**

areas in the figure; B areas are shaded). This is presumably due to either chemotactic factors unique to particular sites, or to recognition of different lymphocytes by local elements such as the inner surface of the vascular endothelium or the dendritic antigen-presenting cells (not shown here, but see Fig. 7).

In general, lymph nodes respond to antigens introduced into the tissues they drain, and the spleen to antigens in the blood. The gut, lungs, breast, and external mucous surfaces also have their own less specialized lymphoid areas which to some extent behave as a separate circuit for recirculation purposes and are often known as the **mucosa-associated lymphoid tissues** or MALT. The same may apply to the skin (SALT). In each case the objective seems to be to provide a local lymphoid system specialized for the antigens most likely to be encountered there.

LYMPH NODE

Lymph nodes (or 'glands') constitute the main bulk of the organized lymphoid tissue. They are strategically placed so that lymph from most parts of the body drains through a series of nodes before reaching the thoracic duct (**TD**), which empties into the left subclavian vein to allow the lymphocytes to recirculate again via the blood.

AL, EL Afferent and efferent lymphatics, through which lymph passes from the tissues to first peripheral and then central lymph nodes.

S Lymphatic sinus, through which lymph flows from the afferent lymphatic into the cortical and medullary sinuses.

M Medullary sinus, collecting lymph for exit via the efferent lymphatic. It is in the medulla that antibody formation takes place and plasma cells are prominent.

G Germinal centre; an area of larger cells that develops within the follicle after antigenic stimulation. It is thought to be the site of B memory-cell generation, and contains special dendritic cells which retain antigens on their surface for weeks and perhaps even years (see Fig. 17 for further details).

T T cell area, or 'paracortex', largely occupied by T cells but through which B cells travel to reach the medulla. It is thought that the dendritic cells here are specialized for presentation of antigen to T cells.

PCV Post-capillary venule; a specialized small venule with high cuboidal endothelium through which lymphocytes leave the blood to enter the paracortex and thence the efferent lymphatic.

SPLEEN

The spleen differs from a lymph node in having no lymphatic drainage, and also in containing large numbers of red cells. In some species it can act as an erythropoietic organ or a reservoir for blood.

TR Trabecula(e); connective tissue structures sheathing the vessels, especially veins.

T T cell area; the lymphoid sheath surrounding the arteries is mostly composed of T lymphocytes.

B B cell area, or lymphoid follicle, typically lying to one side of the lymphoid sheath. Germinal centres are commonly found in the follicle, alongside the follicular artery.

M Marginal zone, the region between the lymphoid areas and the red pulp, where lymphocytes chiefly leave the blood to enter the lymphoid areas, and red cells and plasma cells to enter the red pulp.

RP Red pulp; a reticular meshwork through which blood passes to enter the venous sinusoids, and in which surveillance and removal of damaged red cells is thought to occur. For contrast, the lymphoid areas are sometimes called 'white pulp'. Macrophages in the red pulp and in the marginal zone can retain antigens, as the dendritic cells in the lymph nodes do. As in the medulla of the lymph node, plasma cells are frequent.

S Sinusoids, the large sacs which collect blood for return via the splenic vein.

MUCOSA-ASSOCIATED LYMPHOID TISSUES

Gut The illustration shows a typical Peyer's patch from the ileum, but lymphoid nodules are found up and down the gut, responding to antigens entering through the gut. They are sometimes known collectively as gut-associated lymphoid tissue (GALT), and contain specialized M cells which transport antigens from the lumen into the subepithelial area, where large numbers of lymphocytes are found, particularly of CD8, $\gamma\delta$-receptor T cells. Further in, in the lamina propria, all types of T and B cells are found, particularly IgA B cells, as well as macrophages and mast cells. There are as many lymphocytes in 2 metres of gut as in the whole of the marrow, spleen and lymph nodes.

Lung Like the gut, this is a major site of contact with exogenous antigens, and lymphoid tissue is similarly organized in association with the bronchi (BALT).

Pharynx Lymphoid masses, such as tonsils and adenoids, respond to antigens from the nose and throat. Both B and T cells are present and germinal centres are common. The salivary glands also contain lymphocytes of MALT origin.

Skin Antigens entering via the skin can reach the local lymph node by being taken up in Langerhans cells (**LC** in figure, and see Fig. 7), which can pass from the skin to the node, where they probably settle in the T cell areas. LC are extremely sensitive to UV light, which may be why UV reduces contact sensitivity reactions and conceivably also why it facilitates the induction of suppressor rather than helper T cells (see Fig. 30 for the significance of this in relation to skin cancer).

12 Evolution of recognition molecules

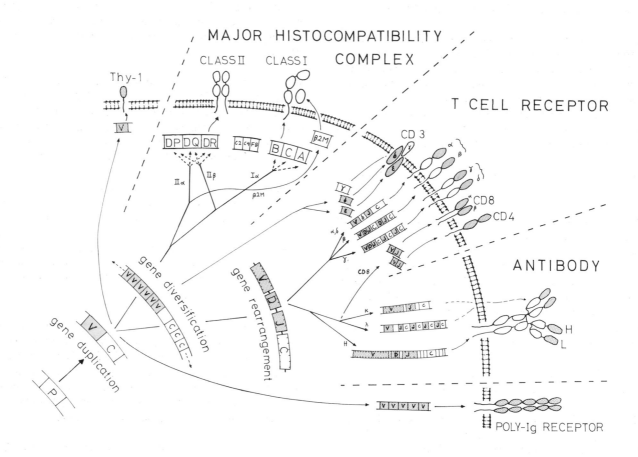

At this point it may be worth re-emphasizing the difference between 'natural' and 'adaptive' immunity, which lies essentially in the degree of **discrimination** of the respective recognition systems.

Natural immune recognition, e.g. by phagocytic cells or the alternative complement pathway, while incompletely understood and extremely interesting, appears to be based on relatively simple distinctions: generally speaking, a particular foreign material is either recognized and dealt with or not: a 'friend or foe' approach.

Recognition by **lymphocytes**, the fundamental cells of adaptive immunity, is quite another matter. An enormous range of foreign substances can be individually distinguished and the appropriate response set in motion. This is only possible because of the evolution of three sets of **cell-surface receptors**, each showing extensive heterogeneity, namely the **antibody** molecule, the **T cell receptor** and the molecules of the **major histocompatibility complex** (MHC). Thanks to

molecular biology, the fascinating discovery has been made that all these receptors share enough sequences, at both the gene (DNA) and protein (amino acid) level, to make it clear that they have evolved from a single precursor, presumably a primitive recognition molecule of some kind (see Fig. 3).

Because antibody was the first of these genetic systems to be identified, they are often collectively referred to as the **immunoglobulin gene superfamily**, which contains other related molecules too, some with immunological functions, some at present without. What they all share is a structure based on a number of folded sequences about 110 amino acids long, called **domains** (shown in the figure as circular loops protruding from the cell membrane).

Much work is still needed to fill in the evolutionary gaps, and the figure can only give an impression of what the relationships between this remarkable family of molecules may have been. Their present-day structure and function are considered in more detail in the following four figures.

P The precursor gene from which the Ig superfamily is presumed to have evolved. It has not been identified in any existing species, but possibly it coded for a self-recognizing molecule such as that used by sponges (see Fig. 3).

V, C A vital early step seems to have been the duplication of this gene into two, one of which became the parent of all present-day **variable** (V) genes and the other of **constant** (C) genes. In the figure the genes and polypeptides with significant enough homology to be considered part of the V gene family are shown shaded. Subsequent further duplications, with diversification among different V and C genes, led ultimately to the large variety of present-day domains.

Thy 1 A molecule of unknown function found on mouse T cells.

Major histocompatibility complex The genes shown are those found in man, also known as HLA (human leucocyte antigen) genes. They code for two types of cell-surface molecule found on all nucleated cells (Class I) or some immunological cells only (Class II). Their α and β chains contain constant regions but it is not certain whether the outer domains are derived from V genes. Interactions between MHC molecules and T cell receptors are vital to all adaptive immune responses.

B2M β2 microglobulin, which combines with Class I chains to complete the four-domain molecule.

C2, C4, FB Three complement components which, rather surprisingly, are coded for by genes lying within the MHC, but are structurally quite unrelated to MHC molecules.

Gene rearrangement A process found only in T and B cells, through which an enormous degree of receptor diversity is generated by bringing together one V gene, one J gene (and one D gene in the case of IgH chains), each from a set containing from two up to several hundred. It involves excisions of DNA and results in a messenger RNA in which further excisions lead to a polypeptide chain composed of only one combination out of the possible thousands. Since a unique gene rearrangement occurs in each T and B cell, and is then inherited in the progeny, each lymphocyte or clone of lymphocytes is effectively unique—which forms the basis for all adaptive immune responses (see Figs 17, 19, 20).

T cell receptor (TCR) A complex of T cell surface molecules, including TCR α plus β, or γ plus δ chains, CD3 and CD4 or CD8, depending on the type of T cell. Together these form a unit which enables the T cell to recognize a specific antigen plus a particular MHC molecule, to become activated and to carry out its function (help, cytotoxicity, etc.)

Antibody The antibody or immunoglobulin molecule plays the part of cell-surface receptor on B lymphocytes as well as being secreted in vast amounts by activated B cells to give rise to serum antibody—a vital part of defence against infectious organisms. The domains are fairly similar to those of the T cell receptor α and β chains, but assembled in a different way, with 2 four-domain heavy (H) chains bonded to 2 two-domain light (L) chains.

Note that the process of diversification in the genes for the various chains has not always proceeded in the same way. For example, mammalian heavy and light (κ) chains have all their J genes together, between V and C, while light (λ) chains have repeated J–C segments and sharks have the whole V–D–J–C segment duplicated—a considerably less efficient arrangement for generating the maximum diversity.

Poly-Ig receptor A molecule found on some epithelial cells which helps to transport antibody into secretions such as mucus. Many other molecules show traces of the characteristic domain structure, including some Fc receptors, adhesion molecules, and receptors for growth factors and cytokines. The common feature seems to be an involvement in cell–cell interactions, with the 'breakaway' immunoglobulin molecule the exception rather than the rule.

13 The major histocompatibility complex

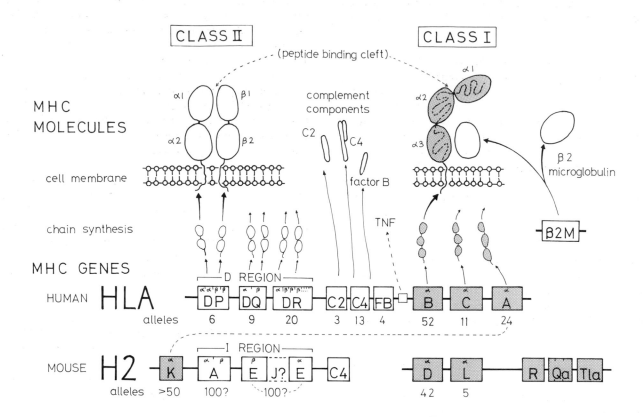

This large and important set of genes owes its rather clumsy-sounding name to the fact that the proteins it codes for were first detected by their effect on transplant rejection. However, it is now clear that their real purpose is to act as 'identity markers' on the surface of the various cells with which T lymphocytes need to interact, via their own receptors, in carrying out their adaptive immunological functions.

Again for historical reasons, the MHC in the mouse (extreme bottom line in the figure) is known as **H-2**, while in man it is called **HLA** ('human leucocyte antigen'). In fact the basic layout of the MHC genes is remarkably similar in all animals so far studied, consisting of a set of Class I (shaded in the figure) and a set of Class II genes, differing slightly in structure and in the way they interact with T cells (see Fig. 14). In the figure the names of genes are

shown boxed, while the numbers below indicate the number of alternative versions or **alleles** which can occur at each locus. Clearly there is enormous polymorphism throughout the whole MHC, and the number of possible combinations on a single chromosome probably exceeds 3×10^6, so that an individual, with a set of MHC molecules coded for by both chromosomes, can have any one of about 10^{13} combinations, which is part of the problem in transplanting kidneys, etc. (see Fig. 36).

Since HLA typing became a routine procedure, it has emerged that many diseases are significantly commoner, or sometimes rarer, in people of a particular HLA type. There are several mechanisms which might account for this but none of them has yet been established to everybody's satisfaction.

H2 The MHC of the mouse, carried on chromosome 17. There are at least 20 other minor histocompatibility genes on other chromosomes, numbered H1, H3, H4 etc: but H2 is by far the strongest in causing transplant rejection and the only one known to be involved in normal cell interactions.

K, D, L The Class I genes of H2, coding for the α chain (MW 44 000), which in combination with β2 microglobulin (see below) makes up the four-domain K, D and L molecules or 'antigens'. The N-terminal portions of the α chains are extremely variable, having probably evolved to interact with different viruses. Because any cell can potentially be infected by a virus, Class I antigens are expressed on virtually all cells in the body, with the exception of red blood cells in some species. The number of different alleles known is shown below each locus, but these are no doubt underestimates.

R, Qa, T1a are also considered part of the Class I family because they code for very similar molecules, but they are expressed only on some lymphocytes and do not mediate transplant rejection. It is suspected that the extensive diversity of the other MHC genes may be generated in this 'Qa region'.

A, E, J The Class II genes of H2, collectively known as the I region. A and E contain separate genes for the α (MW 33 000) and β (MW 28 000) chains of the four-domain molecule. Unlike Class I, Class II molecules are expressed only on a minority of cells, namely those which T cells need to interact with and regulate (see Fig. 14). There are probably more A and E genes than shown in the figure, each with numerous alleles, making a very large number of different antigen recognizing sites on the N-terminal region of the Ia molecule. The status of J is uncertain because although breeding experiments suggest a locus between A and E, coding for products recognized particularly by T suppressor cells, molecular biologists do not find the corresponding DNA in this part of the chromosome.

HLA The human MHC, on chromosome 6, closely analogous to H2 except that the Class I genes lie together.

A, B, C The human Class I genes. A is the homologue of K in the mouse. There are probably Qa and Tla-like genes, not yet characterized.

DP, DQ, DR The human Class II genes. The DP gene product is particularly potent at stimulating T cell proliferation and is tested for by the 'mixed lymphocyte reaction', while all other Class I and II antigens are detected by antibodies made against them. There are other genes (DO, DZ, DX) in this region but it is not clear whether they code for functional molecules. Of the two chains, the β chain appears to contribute almost all the variability, which permits interaction with different antigens and then with the T cell receptor. In general, antigens taken in by the cell and digested in lysosomes become associated with MHC Class II, and those generated within the cell (e.g. by virus) with Class I. How the antigenic fragments 'sit' in the MHC molecule is shown in Fig. 14.

C2, C4, FB These 'Class III' genes all code for complement components involved in the activation of C3. Curiously enough, these exist in several allelic forms, though this has no obvious significance. C4 can become attached to red cells and masquerade as a 'blood group'. Other genes located in this region include those coding for the adrenal enzyme 21-hydroxylase and for the cytokines TNFα and β.

B2M β2 microglobulin, (MW 12 000) coded quite separately from the MHC, nevertheless forms part of all Class I molecules, stabilizing them on the cell surface. In the mouse there are two allelic forms, but in general β2M is one of the most remarkably conserved molecules known. It is also found free in the serum.

HLA-ASSOCIATED DISEASES

The most remarkable example is the rare sleep abnormality narcolepsy, which virtually only occurs in people carrying the DR2 antigen; the reason is quite unknown. After this, the most striking example is the group of arthropathies involving the sacroiliac joint (ankylosing spondylitis, Reiter's disease, etc.) where one HLA allele (B27) is found in up to 95% of cases—nearly 20 times its frequency in the general population. But numerous other diseases, including almost all of the autoimmune diseases, show a statistically significant association with particular HLA antigens or groups of antigens, especially in the D region. The tendency of HLA alleles (for example A1 and B8) to 'stay together' instead of segregating normally is called 'linkage disequilibrium' and may imply that such combinations are of survival value, perhaps because they increase resistance to diseases or, alternatively, because they reduce the risk of hypersensitivity. This whole field is still in an exciting stage of evolution.

14 The T cell receptor

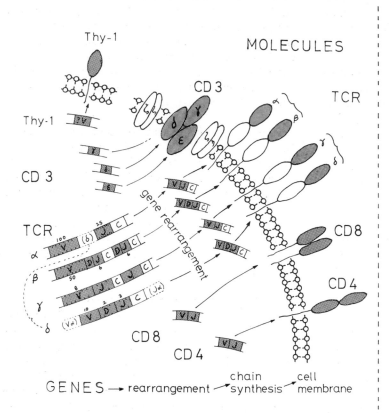

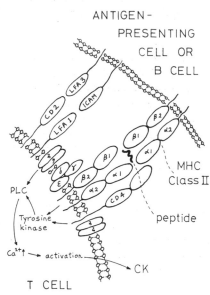

INTERACTION BETWEEN A CD4αβ
HELPER T CELL, A FOREIGN
PEPTIDE, AND AN MHC MOLECULE

It has been evident for many years that T lymphocytes have a surface receptor for antigen, with roughly similar properties to the antibody on B lymphocytes, but furious controversy raged as to whether the two molecules were in fact identical. The issue was finally resolved in 1983–4 by the use of monoclonal antibodies to study the fine structure of the molecule and of DNA probing to identify the corresponding genes, and it is now clear that the T cell receptor is a quite separate entity.

Like all members of the immunoglobulin superfamily, the T cell receptor has a structure of polypeptide chains made up of domains, linked together by disulphide bonds. In this case there are two major chains (α, β) each of two domains, but other molecules (e.g. CD3, CD4, CD8) also play a role in T cell interactions with MHC molecules, and a second (γδ) combination is found on some T cells instead of αβ. The way in which the T cell receptor 'recognizes' a foreign antigen in association with an MHC molecule is illustrated in the right-hand part of the figure; in this case the T cell is

of the helper variety. Knowledge of these interactions is far from complete, but advances should be rapid now that the long-awaited breakthrough has been made.

An unusual feature of these proteins is that the genes for different parts of each polypeptide chain do not lie together on the chromosome, so that unwanted segments of DNA, and subsequently of RNA, have to be excised to bring them together. This process is known as **gene rearrangement** and occurs only in T cells, so that in all other cells the genes remain in their non-functional 'germ line' configuration. Once this rearrangement has occurred in an individual T lymphocyte, that cell is committed to a unique receptor, and therefore a unique antigen-recognizing ability. A similar thing happens to the immunoglobulin genes in B cells (see Fig. 15). In this and the following figure, the portions of genes and proteins which are shaded are those thought to have evolved from the primitive V region, though they do not all show the same degree of variability.

TCR The T cell receptor. It is made up of one α (MW 50 000) and one β (MW 45 000) chain, each with an outer variable domain, an inner constant domain and short intramembrane and cytoplasmic regions. Some T cells, especially early in foetal life and in some organs like the gut and skin, express the alternative γδ receptor and seem to recognize a different set of antigens from the αβ population.

CD3 A complex of three chains, γ (MW 25 000), δ (MW 20 000), and ε (MW 20 000) which is essential to all T cell function. Also associated with the TCR–CD3 complex are other two-chain signalling molecules known as ζζ and ζη. Interaction of antigen (i.e. MHC-plus-peptide) with this whole complex leads to cell activation via at least two intracellular pathways, involving tyrosine kinase and phospholipase C, which eventually lead to proliferation and cytokine release.

CD4 A single-domain molecule (MW 60 000) found on human helper T cells. It is involved in the interaction with MHC Class II molecules (as shown in the figure). The equivalent in the mouse is known as L3T4. CD4 is the 'receptor' by which the AIDS virus enters T cells. (See Fig. 39.)

CD8 A 75 000 MW molecule found on most cytotoxic and suppressor T cells. In man it is composed of two identical chains, but the equivalent in the mouse has two different chains (Ly2/3). It is involved in interacting with MHC Class I molecules. Both CD4 and CD8 are linked to the intracellular signalling pathway but the details remain to be worked out.

Thy 1 A single-domain molecule found on mouse T cells and also on some brain cells. Its function is not known, but there are also other members of the immunoglobulin superfamily in the brain, which may have a recognition role in neurological pathways.

Gene rearrangement The TCR genes contain up to 100 V genes and numerous J genes, so that to make a single chain, one of each must be linked up to the correct C gene. This is done by excision of intervening DNA sequences and further excision in the messenger RNA, eventually producing a single V–D–J–C in RNA to code for the polypeptide chain. When all the possible combinations of α and β chains are taken into account, the number of different TCR molecules available to an individual may be as high as 10^{10}. Note that the CD4 and CD8 genes, though apparently of V gene origin, do not rearrange and the molecules therefore do not show such diversity.

Antigen Shown in the figure as a short peptide, in this case being 'recognized' by an MHC molecule and the T cell receptor. If this recognition is strong enough, aided by CD4-MHC interaction, the CD3 molecule will undergo changes which lead to an increase in intracellular calcium and probably other ion movements. The T cell is then **activated** to carry out its programmed function. In the case of a cytotoxic T cell, a CD8 molecule would play the part of CD4, by interacting with MHC Class I molecules on the cell to be killed.

CK Cytokines, the principal secreted product of T cells, with effects on many other cells such as B lymphocytes, macrophages, eosinophils, etc. (see Fig. 22). It is not known precisely how the nature of the activating signal influences which cytokine is produced, but experiments with cloned T cells, especially in mice, suggest that some CD4 T cells (TH1) make mainly IFNγ and other cytokines involved in activating macrophages, while others (TH2) make predominantly the antibody-helper factors IL4, IL5, IL6, etc. In man, however, this distinction is less clear.

LFA, ICAM, CD2 Other surface molecules on T cells and/or antigen-presenting cells, which interact to increase the overall affinity of cell–cell interaction. They are collectively known as adhesion molecules.

15 Antibody diversification and synthesis

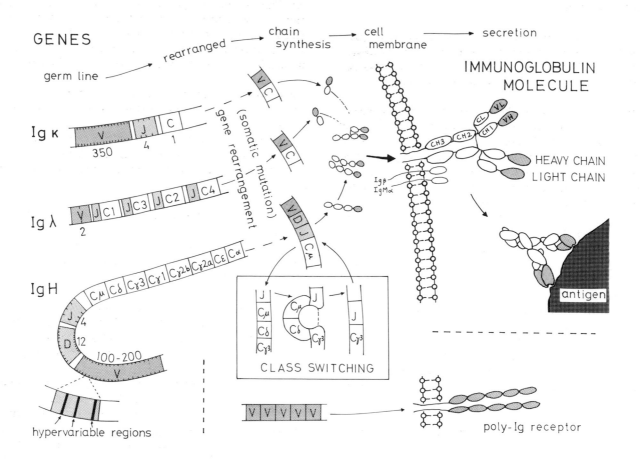

In contrast to the MHC and the T cell receptor, the existence of the antibody, or **immunoglobulin** (Ig) molecule has been known for 100 years and its basic structure for about 30, which makes it one of the most studied and best understood molecules in biology.

The two-chain multi-domain structure characteristic of MHC and T cell receptors is seen here in a slightly different form, a typical Ig molecule being made up of four chains—a pair of **heavy** chains and a pair of **light chains** (see Fig. 16 for structural details). Two main kinds of diversity are found within these chains: in the **constant** regions of the heavy chains are the variations which classify Ig molecules into classes and subclasses with different biological effects, while the much more extensive variations in the **variable** regions (shaded in the figure) are responsible for the shape of the antigen-binding site and thus of the antigen specificity of the Ig molecule.

Within B lymphocytes, the genes for Ig heavy and light chains are put together by a process of rearrangement at the DNA level followed by further excisions in the messenger RNA, very much as in T cells with their receptor. Finally, the polypeptide chains are synthesized on ribosomes like other proteins, assembled and exported—some to reside on the cell surface as receptors and others to be secreted into the blood as antibody.

Ig Immunoglobulin; the name given to all globulins with antibody activity. It has replaced the old term 'gamma globulin' because not all antibodies have gamma electrophoretic mobility.

Igκ, Igλ, IgH Three genetic loci on different chromosomes which code for the light chain (κ, λ) and heavy (H) chain of the Ig molecule. A typical Ig molecule has two H chains and two L chains—either both κ or both λ.

Germ line This denotes those genes in the ova and sperm giving rise to successive generations, which can be regarded as a continuous family tree stretching back to the earliest forms of life. Mutations and other genetic changes in these genes are passed to subsequent generations and are what natural selection works on. Changes which occur in any other cells of the body are 'somatic' and affect only the individual, being lost when he dies. This includes the changes in the DNA of B lymphocytes which lead to the formation of the Ig molecule. The antibody germ-line genes have presumably been selected as indispensable, and many of them have been shown to code for antibodies against common bacteria, confirming that bacterial infection was probably the main stimulus for the evolution of antibody.

V Variable region genes. Their number ranges from two (mouse λ chain) to about 350 (mouse κ chain). The greatest variation is found in three short **hypervariable** regions, which code for the amino acids which form the combining site and make contact with the antigen.

C Constant region genes. In the light chains, these code for a single domain only, but in the heavy chains there are three or four domains, numbered CH 1, 2, 3, (4). Which of the eight (mouse) or nine (human) C genes is in use by a particular B lymphocyte determines the class and subclass of the resulting Ig molecule (IgM, IgG, etc., see Fig. 16).

J Joining region genes, coding for the short J segment. Note that in the κ and H chains, the different J genes lie together while in the λ chain each C gene has its own. In primitive vertebrates there are repeated V–J–C segments, which restricts the number of possible combinations.

D Region genes are found only on IgH, where they provide additional possibilities for hypervariability.

Gene rearrangement occurs in the Ig genes of B lymphocytes in a similar way to the TCR genes of T lymphocytes. First the intervening segments of DNA ('introns') between the V and J (and D if present) genes are excised in such a way as to bring together one particular V and one J gene. This is then transcribed to RNA and the segment between this V(D)J segment and the C region are excised, to leave an mRNA able to code for a complete V(D)JC chain.

Class switching can occur within the individual B cell by further excisions of DNA which allow the same VDJ segment to lie next to a different C gene, leading to antibodies with the same specificity for antigen but a different constant region (see Fig. 16). This allows the same antigen to be subjected to various different forms of attack.

Poly-Ig receptor This molecule, found in secretory epithelial cells, allows the transport of Ig into secretions such as mucus, milk and bile. It has recently been found to be composed of V-like domains, emphasizing the wide range of functions within the Ig superfamily.

Origins of diversity Four features of antibody contribute to the enormous number of possible antigen-binding sites, and thus of antibody specificities: (1) gene rearrangement allows any V, D and J genes to become associated; (2) a heavy chain can pair with either a κ or λ light chain; (3) V–D and D–J joining is not always at precisely the same point; (4) mutations can occasionally occur in the V genes of an individual B cell (this would be a case of **somatic mutation**) and the resulting small change in the antigen-binding site may sometimes prove advantageous, e.g. by increasing the affinity of an antibody for the inducing antigen. Because of all these possibilities it is difficult to put a number on the size of the Ig repertoire, but it probably exceeds 10^8. Note that diversity within the MHC is generated in a quite different way, individuals having only one or two of the allelic variants of each gene. Thus the members of a species differ from each other much more in their MHC genes and molecules than in their Ig and T cell receptors, of which they all have a fairly complete set with only minor inherited differences.

Ig-β, IgM-α Two recently discovered molecules that form a dimer that links cell-surface Ig (usually IgM) to intracellular signalling pathways.

16 Antibody structure and function

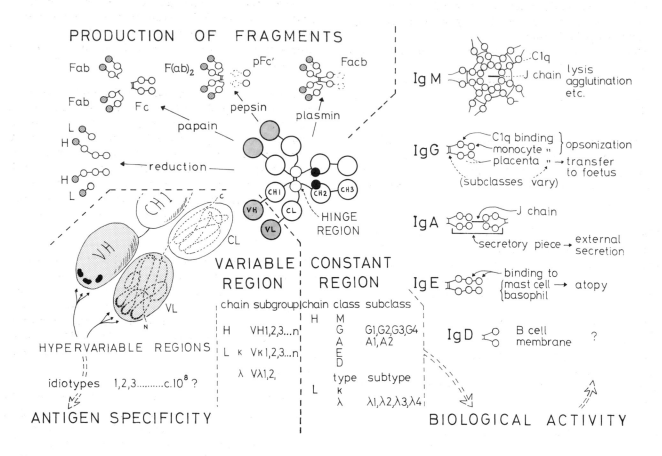

PRODUCTION OF FRAGMENTS

Fab · F(ab)₂ · pFc' · Facb

Fab · Fc · pepsin · plasmin

papain

L · H · reduction · H · L

CH1 · C · CL · VH · VL · CL · HINGE REGION

VARIABLE REGION · CONSTANT REGION

VH · VL

HYPERVARIABLE REGIONS

chain	subgroup	chain	class	subclass
H	VH1,2,3...n	H	M	
L κ	Vκ1,2,3...n		G	G1,G2,G3,G4
			A	A1,A2
λ	Vλ1,2,		E	
			D	
			type	subtype
		L	κ	
			λ	λ1,λ2,λ3,λ4

idiotypes 1,2,3.........c.10^8 ?

ANTIGEN SPECIFICITY

IgM — C1q — J chain — lysis agglutination etc.

IgG — C1q binding / monocyte " / placenta " → opsonization, transfer to foetus (subclasses vary)

IgA — J chain — secretory piece → external secretion

IgE — binding to {mast cell → atopy / basophil}

IgD — B cell membrane — ?

BIOLOGICAL ACTIVITY

Considering that the antibody in serum is a mixture of perhaps 100 million slightly different types of molecule, the unravelling of its structure was no mean feat. Early work depended on separation into fragments by chemical treatment (top left in figure); the fine details have come from amino acid sequencing and X-ray crystallography, both of which require the use of completely homogeneous (monoclonal) antibody. This was originally available only in the form of myeloma proteins, the product of malignant B lymphocytes, but is produced nowadays by the hybridoma method (see Fig. 9).

A typical antibody molecule (IgG, centre) has 12 domains, arranged in two heavy and two light (H and L) chains, linked through cysteine residues by disulphide bonds so that the domains lie together in pairs, the whole molecule having the shape of a flexible **Y**. In each chain the N-terminal domain is the most **variable**, the rest being relatively **constant**. Within the variable (V) regions, the maximum variation in amino acid sequence is seen in the six **hypervariable** regions (three per chain) which come together to form the **antigen-binding site** (bottom left in figure). The constant (C) regions vary mainly in those portions which interact with complement or various cell-surface receptors; the right-hand part of the figure shows the different features of the C region in the five **classes** of antibody; M, G, A, E and D. The result is a huge variety of molecules able to bring any antigen into contact with any one of several effective disposal mechanisms. The basic structure (MW, about 160 000) can form dimers (IgA, MW 400 000) or pentamers (IgM, MW 900 000; see right-hand side of figure).

There are species differences, especially in the heavy chain subclasses, which have evolved comparatively recently; the examples shown here illustrate human antibodies. Attention has recently been focused on the carbohydrate side chains (shown here in black) which may constitute up to 12% of the whole molecule. They are thought to be associated mainly with secretion, but are abnormal in certain diseases.

Note The illustration shows an IgG molecule with its 12 domains stylized. The actual 3-dimensional structure is more like the molecule shown binding to antigen in Fig. 15 (extreme right).

Fragments   produced by chemical treatment:

H, L: Heavy and light chains which, being only disulphide-linked, separate under reducing conditions.

Fab: antigen-binding fragment (papain digestion).

Fc: crystallizable (because relatively homogeneous fragment). (papain digestion.)

F(ab): two Fab fragments united by disulphide bonds (pepsin digestion).

pFc: a dimer of CH3 domains (pepsin digestion).

Facb: an Ig molecule lacking CH3 domains (plasmin digestion).

Chains   The heavy and two types of light (κ, λ) chains are coded for by genes on different chromosomes, but sequence homologies suggest that all Ig domains originated from a common 'precursor' molecule about 110 amino acids long (see Fig. 12).

Classes   Physical, antigenic and functional variations between constant regions define the five main classes of heavy chain: M, G, A, E and D. These are different molecules, all of which are present in all members of most higher species. Brief points of interest are listed below.

IgM   is usually the first class of antibody made in a response and is also thought to have been the first to appear during evolution (see Fig. 3). Because its pentameric structure gives it up to 10 antigen-combining sites, it is extremely efficient at binding and agglutinating micro-organisms.

IgG   a later development which owes its value to the ability of its Fc portion to bind avidly to C1q (see Fig. 5) and to receptors on phagocytic cells (see Fig. 8). It also gains access to the extravascular spaces and (via the placenta) to the foetus. In most species, IgG has become further diversified into subclasses (see below).

IgA   is the major antibody of secretions such as tears, sweat and the contents of lungs, gut, urine, etc., where, thanks to its secretory piece (see below), it avoids digestion. Its main value is to block the entry of micro-organisms from these external surfaces to the tissues themselves.

IgE   is a curious molecule whose main property is to bind to mast cells and promote their degranulation. The desirable and undesirable consequences of this are discussed in Fig. 32.

IgD   appears to function only on the surface of B cells, where it may have some regulatory role. In the mouse it is unusual in having two instead of three constant regions in the heavy chain.

Subclasses, subtypes, subgroups   Within classes, smaller variations between constant regions define the subclasses found in different molecules of all members of an individual species. The IgG subclasses are generally the most varied. Light chain C region variants of this kind are sometimes called 'subtypes' and those in the V regions 'subgroups'. All these variants found in all individuals of a species are called 'isotypic'. Different IgG subclasses tend to be induced by different types of antigen (e.g. in man, IgG1 and 3 by viruses, IgG2 by carbohydrates) but nobody really knows why this is.

Allotypes   By contrast, 'allotypic' variations (not shown in the figure) distinguish the Ig molecules of some individuals from others (cf. the blood groups). They are genetically determined or perhaps regulated, and occur mainly in the C regions. No biological function has yet been discovered. Unlike blood groups, etc., Ig allotypes are expressed singly on individual B cells, a process known as 'allelic exclusion', which shows that only one of the cell's two sets of chromosomes are used for making antibody—presumably the first one to successfully rearrange its Ig genes.

Hypervariable regions   Three parts of each of the variable regions of heavy and light chains, spaced roughly equally apart in the amino acid sequence (see figure, lower left) but brought close together as the chain folds into a β-pleated sheet, form the antigen-combining site. It is because of the enormous degree of variation in the DNA coding for these regions that the total number of combinations is so high.

Idiotypes   In many cases, antibody molecules with different antigen-combining sites can in turn be distinguished by other antibodies made against them. The latter are known as 'anti-idiotypic', implying that each combining site is associated with a different shape, though this is not always the antigen-binding site itself. Anti-idiotypic antibodies are thought to be formed normally and may help to regulate immune responses (see Fig. 21).

Hinge region   Both flexibility and proteolytic digestion are facilitated by the repeated proline residues in this part of the molecule. In IgM, the hinge region is as large as a normal domain, and is called CH2, so that the other two constant region domains are called CH3 and CH4; the same may be true for IgE.

J chain   A glycopeptide molecule which aids polymerization of IgA and IgM.

Secretory piece   A polypeptide produced in epithelial cells and added to IgA dimers to enable them to be transported across the epithelium and secreted into gut, tears, milk, etc.; where IgA predominates.

C1q   The first component of the classical complement sequence, a hexavalent glycoprotein activated by binding to CH2 domains of IgM and some IgG subclasses (in the human, IgG1 and IgG3).

17 The antibody response

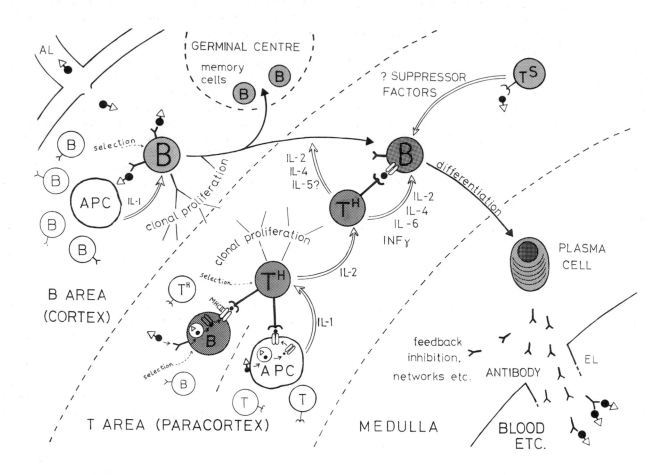

Animals born and reared in the complete absence of contact with any non-self material (not an easy procedure!) have virtually no immunoglobulins in their serum, but as soon as they encounter the normal environment, with its content of bacteria etc., their serum immunoglobulin (Ig) rises towards the normal level of 10–20 mg (or about 60 000 000 000 000 000 molecules) per ml. This shows that immunoglobulins are produced only as a result of stimulation by foreign antigens, the process being known as the **antibody response**.

In the figure, these events are shown in a section through a stylized lymph node. Antigen is shown entering from the tissues (top left) and antibody being released into the blood (bottom right). The antigen is depicted as a combination of two components, representing the portion, or **determinant**, recognized by the B cell and against which antibody is eventually made (black circles) and other determinants which interact with T cells and are needed in order for the B cell to the fully triggered (white triangles). These are usually known as 'haptenic' and 'carrier' determinants respectively. In practice, a virus, bacterium, etc. would carry numerous different haptenic and carrier determinants, whereas small molecules such as

toxins may act as haptens only. But even small, well-defined antigenic determinants usually stimulate a heterogeneous population of B cells, each producing antibody of slightly different specificity and affinity.

The main stages of the response are **presentation** of the antigen, **selection** of the appropriate individual B and T cells (shown shaded), **proliferation** of these cells to form a **clone** and **differentiation** into the mature **functioning** state. A prominent feature of all stages is the many **interactions** between cells which are mediated mostly by cytokines (white arrows in the figure). There are also a number of regulatory influences whose relative importance is not yet clear. Most of these cell interactions occur in the lymph nodes or spleen, but antibody can be formed wherever there is lymphoid tissue.

In a subsequent response to the same antigen, average affinity tends to be higher, precursor T and B cells more numerous and Ig class more varied. This **secondary** response is therefore more rapid and effective, and such an individual is described as showing **memory** to the antigen in question; this, for example, is the aim of most vaccines (see Fig. 40).

AL Afferent lymphatic, via which antigens enter the lymph node (see Fig. 11).

APC Antigen-presenting cell. Before they can trigger lymphocytes, antigens normally require to be presented on the surface of a specialized cell. Various dendritic cells in lymphoid tissue, Langerhans cells in the skin, etc. (see Fig. 7) perform this function, part of which consists of releasing Interleukin-1 (IL-1) (see below) but which in the case of T lymphocytes also requires the presence of Class II MHC molecules on the APC. Except with small peptides that can associate directly with MHC, antigens have to be processed first, by enzyme cleavage within lysosomes.

MAC Macrophages can also present antigen to T and probably B cells, and it has been found recently that B cells themselves have antigen-presenting ability too, but in this case the only cells that can take up and process antigen are those whose surface Ig recognizes it. Thus B cells become relatively more important as presenters when there are more of them with the right specificity, e.g. during secondary responses.

Selection Only a small minority of lymphocytes will recognize and bind to a particular antigen. These lymphocytes are thus 'selected' by the antigen. The binding 'receptor' is surface Ig in the case of the B cell, and the TCR complex in the case of the T cell, which recognizes both antigen and MHC (see Fig. 14).

Clonal proliferation Once selected, lymphocytes divide repeatedly to form a 'clone' of identical cells. The stimulus for this is mainly a soluble product of the APC known as **IL-1** but T cell-derived cytokines are also required for B cell proliferation. T cell proliferation is greatly augmented by another soluble factor (**IL-2**) made by T cells themselves. (For more information on interleukins see Fig. 22.)

Differentiation Once they have proliferated, B cells become susceptible to helper factors from T helper (T^H) cells. Those that have been identified have been given 'interleukin' numbers but almost all the known cytokines have some effect in promoting B cell growth or function. However, certain large repeating antigens can do this without T cell help; they are called 'T independent' and are usually bacterial polysaccharides. As a rule they only stimulate IgM, probably representing a more primitive form of response.

Plasma cell In order to make and secrete antibody, endoplasmic reticulum and ribosomes are developed, giving the B cell its basophilic excentric appearance. Plasma cells can release up to 2000 antibody molecules per second, but they only live for a few days.

EL Efferent lymphatic, via which antibody formed in the medulla reaches the lymph and eventually the blood for distribution to all parts of the body.

Memory cells Instead of differentiating into antibody-producing plasma cells, some B cells persist as memory cells, whose increased number and rapid response underlies the highly augmented secondary response, essentially a faster and larger version of the primary response, starting out from more of the appropriate B (and T^H) cells. Memory B cells differ slightly from their precursors (more surface Ig, more likely to recirculate in the blood) but retain the same specificity for antigen. The generation of memory B cells appears to take place in **germinal centres** and to require the presence of complement. It is also somehow linked to T cells, since T independent responses do not usually show memory. T^H cells also develop into memory cells but their precise location is not known.

TS T suppressor cells are also stimulated during most antibody responses, especially when antigen is not presented by APC. They may be specific for hapten (as shown in the figure), for carrier determinants (in which case they inhibit the T helper cells), or for the idiotypic B or T receptors, or they may be non-specific, suppressing all responses in their immediate vicinity. Like help, suppression is probably carried out by soluble factors, though the whole subject is very controversial (see Fig. 20).

Feedback inhibition Antibody itself, particularly IgG, can inhibit its own formation, partly by eliminating the antigen, but perhaps also by stimulating T suppressor cells.

Networks It was hypothesized by Jerne, and subsequently shown, that antibody idiotypes (i.e. the unique portions related to specificity) can themselves act as antigens, and promote both B and T cell responses against the cells carrying them, so that the immune response progressively damps itself out. This leads to the fascinating concept of a network of anti-idiotype receptors corresponding to all the antigens an animal can respond to—a sort of 'internal image' of its external environment (see Fig. 21 for a further discussion). However, the actual role of networks in regulating ordinary antibody responses is not yet clear, nor is that of suppressor T cells. In practice the single most important element in regulating antibody production is probably the removal of the antigen itself.

18 Antigen–antibody interaction and immune complexes

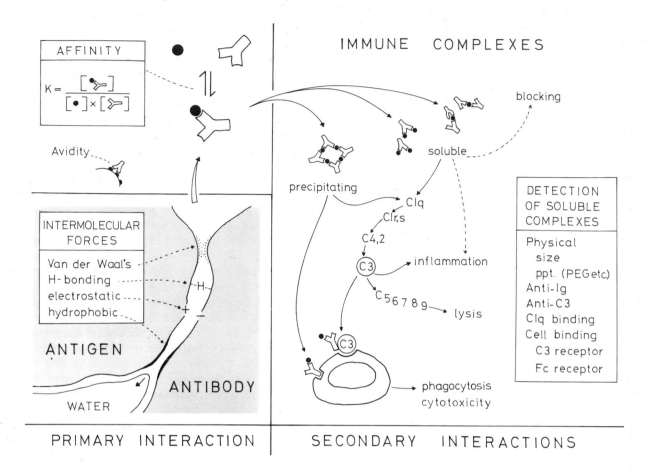

AFFINITY

$$K = \frac{[\,\multimap\!\bullet\,]}{[\,\bullet\,] \times [\,\multimap\,]}$$

Avidity

INTERMOLECULAR FORCES

Van der Waal's
H-bonding
electrostatic
hydrophobic

ANTIGEN

ANTIBODY

WATER

PRIMARY INTERACTION

IMMUNE COMPLEXES

blocking

soluble

precipitating

C1q
C1r,s
C4,2
C3 → inflammation
C56789 → lysis

C3 → phagocytosis
cytotoxicity

DETECTION OF SOLUBLE COMPLEXES

Physical
 size
 ppt. (PEG etc)
Anti-Ig
Anti-C3
C1q binding
Cell binding
 C3 receptor
 Fc receptor

SECONDARY INTERACTIONS

An antigen, by definition, stimulates the production of antibody, which in turn combines with the antigen. Both processes are based on **complementarity** (or 'fit') between two **shapes**—a small piece of the antigen (or **determinant**) and the **combining site** of the antibody, a cleft formed largely by the hypervariable regions of heavy and light chains (see Fig. 16). The closer the fit between this site and the antigenic determinant, the stronger will be the non-covalent forces (hydrophobic, electrostatic, etc., lower left) between them, and the higher the **affinity** (top left). When both combining sites can interact with the same antigen (e.g. on a cell), the bond has a greatly increased strength, which in this case is referred to as 'avidity'.

The ability of a particular antibody to combine with one determinant rather than another is referred to as **specificity**. The antibody repertoire of an animal, stored in its V genes (see Fig. 15), is expressed as the number of different shapes towards which a complementary specific antibody molecule can be made, and runs into millions.

What happens when antigen and antibody combine depends on the circumstances. Sometimes antibody alone is enough to neutralize the antigen, as in the case of those toxins or micro-organisms which need to attach to cell surface receptors in order to gain entry; antibody can often block this.

Usually however, a secondary interaction of the antibody molecule with another effector agent, such as complement or phagocytic cells, is required to dispose of the antigen. The importance of these secondary interactions is shown by the fact that deficiency of complement or myeloid cells can be almost as serious as deficiency of antibody itself (see Fig. 38).

The combination of antigen and antibody is called an **immune complex**; this may be small (soluble) or large (precipitating), depending on the nature and proportions of antigen and antibody (top right). The usual fate of complexes is to be removed by phagocytic cells, through the interaction of the Fc portion of the antibody with complement and with cell-surface receptors (bottom centre and Fig. 8). However, in some cases complexes may persist in circulation and cause inflammatory damage to organs (see Fig. 33) or inhibit useful immunity, e.g. to tumours or parasites. The detection of complexes and the identification of the antigen in them is therefore important and numerous techniques are available.

ANTIGEN–ANTIBODY INTERACTION

The combining site of antibody is a cleft roughly $3 \times 1 \times 1$ nm (the size of five or six sugar units), though there is evidence that antigens may bind to larger, or even separate, parts of the variable region. Binding depends on a close 3-dimensional fit, allowing weak intermolecular forces to overcome the normal repulsion between molecules.

Van der Waal's forces attract all molecules through their electron clouds, but only act at extremely close range.

Hydrogen bonding, e.g. between $-NH_2$ and $-OH$ groups, is another weak force.

Electrostatic attraction between antibody and antigen molecules with a net opposite charge is sometimes quite strong.

Hydrophobic regions on antigen and antibody will tend to be attracted in an aqueous environment; this is probably the strongest force between them.

Affinity is normally expressed as the association constant under equilibrium conditions. A value of 10^3 litres/mole would be considered low, while high affinity antibody can reach 10^{10} litres/mole and over—several orders of magnitude higher than most enzyme-substrate interactions. In practice, it is often **avidity** which is measured because antibodies have (at least) two valencies, and even with monovalent antigens a serum can only be assigned an average affinity. Average affinity tends to increase with time after antigenic stimulation, partly through cell selection by diminishing amounts of antigen, and partly via somatic mutation of Ig genes. High affinity antibodies are more effective in most cases, but low affinity antibodies persist too, and may have certain advantages (re-usability, resistance to tolerance?).

IMMUNE COMPLEXES

Under conditions of antigen or antibody excess, small ('soluble') complexes tend to predominate, but with roughly equivalent amounts of antigen and antibody, precipitates form, probably by lattice formation. In the presence of complement (i.e. in fresh serum) only small complexes are formed; in fact C3 can actually solubilize larger complexes (see also Fig. 33).

Blocking of T cell or antibody-mediated killing by complexes in (respectively) antigen or antibody excess, may account for some of the unresponsiveness to tumours or parasite infections.

C1q the first component of complement, binds to the Fc portion of complexed antibody, possibly under the influence of a conformational change in the shape of the Ig molecule, although some workers hold that occupation of both combining sites (i.e. of IgG) is all that is needed. Activation of the 'classical' complement pathway follows.

Inflammation Breakdown products of C3 and C5, through interaction with mast cells, polymorphs, etc., are responsible for the vascular damage which is a feature of 'immune complex diseases' (see Fig. 33).

Lysis, e.g. of bacteria, requires the complete complement sequence. Sometimes the C567 unit moves away from the original site of antibody binding, activates C8 and 9, and causes lysis of innocent cells, (e.g. red cells); this is known as 'reactive lysis'.

Phagocytosis by macrophages, polymorphs, eosinophils, etc. is the normal fate of large complexes. In general, the antibody classes and subclasses which bind to Fc receptors also bind to complement, making them strongly opsonic, but the Fc and C3 receptors are quite distinct; IgM, for example, binds to complement much more than to cells.

Cytotoxicity When antibody bound to a cell or micro-organism makes contact with Fc receptors, the result may be killing rather than phagocytosis. Cells able to do this include macrophages, monocytes, neutrophils, eosinophils, and the lymphocyte-like 'K' cell (see Fig. 9). The importance of this type of 'antibody-mediated cytotoxicity' *in vivo* is controversial.

Detection of soluble complexes

Complexes tend to be of large size (e.g. in the ultracentrifuge or gradients), and to precipitate in the cold ('cryoprecipitation') and in polyethylene glycol (PEG). Since they contain Ig, complexes react with anti-Ig antibodies (e.g. rheumatoid factor). Their reaction with C1q is used in a number of sensitive assays, and the presence of C3 can be deduced from reaction with anti-C3 antibody (immunoconglutinin) and binding to cells with C3 receptors, such as the Raji cell line. In general, these assays agree, but some complexes do not fix complement yet are precipitated by PEG, while some tests can be complicated by the presence of other large molecules. Therefore several tests may need to be done in parallel.

CENTRAL NERVOUS SYSTEM

Cortex The outer layer of the brain in which conscious sensations, language, thought, and memory are controlled.

Limbic system An intermediate zone responsible for the more emotional aspects of behaviour.

Hypothalamus The innermost part of the limbic system, which regulates not only behaviour and mood but also vital physical functions such as food and water intake and temperature, It has connections to and from the cortex, brain stem, and endocrine system.

Pituitary gland The 'conductor of the endocrine orchestra', a gland about the size of a pea, divided into anterior and posterior portions secreting different hormones (see below).

RH Specific releasing hormones produced in the hypothalamus stimulate the pituitary to release its own hormones (e.g. TRH, TSH-releasing hormone).

Neuropeptides Small molecules responsible for some of the transmission of signals in the CNS. The hypothalamus produces several that cause pain (e.g. substance P) or suppress it (e.g. endorphins, encephalins).

AUTONOMIC NERVOUS SYSTEM

In general, **sympathetic** nerves, via the secretion of noradrenaline, (epinephrine), excite functions involved in urgent action ('fight or flight') such as cardiac output, respiration, blood sugar, awareness, sweating.

Parasympathetic nerves, many of which travel via cranial nerve **X** (the vagus), secrete acetylcholine and promote more peaceful activities such as digestion and close vision. Most viscera are regulated by one or the other or both. Massive sympathetic activation (including the adrenal medulla, see below), is triggered by fear, rage, etc.—the 'alarm' reaction which if allowed to become chronic, shades over into **stress**.

ENDOCRINE SYSTEM

Adrenal medulla The inner part of the adrenal gland, which when stimulated by sympathetic nerves releases **adrenaline**, with effects similar to noradrenaline but more prolonged.

Adrenal cortex The outer part of the adrenal gland, stimulated by corticotrophin (ACTH) from the anterior pituitary to secrete aldosterone, hydrocortisone (cortisol) and other hormones that regulate salt/water balance and protein and carbohydrate metabolism. In addition hydrocortisone and its synthetic derivatives have powerful anti-inflammatory effects.

Thyroid Stimulated by thyrotrophin (TSH) from the anterior pituitary to release the iodine-containing thyroid hormones T3 and T4 (thyroxine) which regulate many aspects of cellular metabolism.

Growth hormone (GH) regulates the size of bones and soft tissues.

Gonads Two anterior pituitary hormones, follicle-stimulating (FSH) and luteinizing (LH) regulate the development of testes and ovaries, puberty, and the release of sex hormones. These changes are especially subject to hypothalamic influence—e.g. psychic, or, in animals, seasonal.

Posterior pituitary Here the main product is anti-diuretic hormone (ADH), which retains water via the kidneys in response to osmotic receptors in the hypothalamus.

The **pancreas** and **parathyroids** function more or less autonomously to regulate glucose and calcium levels respectively, although the pancreas also responds to autonomic nervous signals.

IMMUNE SYSTEM

(*Note*: the elements shown in the figure are all considered in detail elsewhere in this book. Here, attention is drawn only to the features linking them to the nervous and endocrine systems.)

Cytokines The most convincing immune–nervous system link is the induction of fever by TNF, IL-1, IFNs; high doses of many cytokines also cause drowsiness and general malaise. Cytokines, especially IL-2 and IL-6, are found in the brain. TNF and IL-1 are thought to induce ACTH secretion from the pituitary, probably via the hypothalamus.

Lymphoid organs Neurons terminating in the thymus and lymph nodes can be traced via sympathetic nerves to the spinal cord.

Lymphocytes have been shown to bear receptors for endorphins, encephalins and substance P, and also to secrete endorphins and hormones such as ACTH.

Immune responses are inhibited by hydrocortisone and sex hormones, and under stressful conditions, particularly when stress is inescapable, as with bereavement, examinations, etc. Whether corticosteroids can explain all such cases is a hotly debated point.

Autoimmunity It is remarkable how many autoimmune diseases (see Fig. 35) affect endocrine organs. Especially striking is the thyroid, where autoantibodies can both mimic and block the stimulating effect of TSH.

24 Anti-microbial immunity: a general scheme

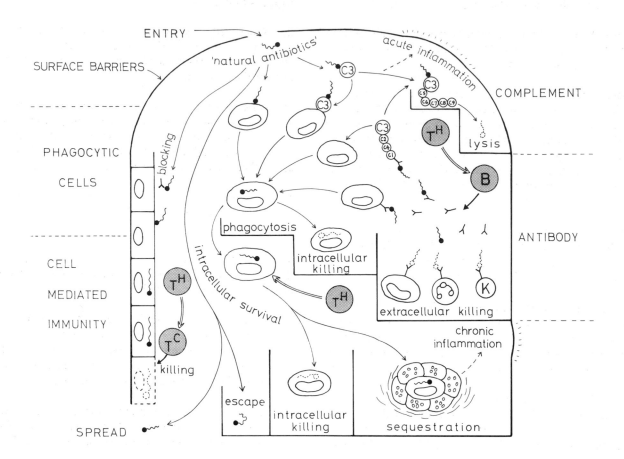

At this point the reader will appreciate that the immune system is highly efficient at recognizing **foreign** substances by their shape but has no infallible way of distinguishing whether or not they are **dangerous**. By and large, this approach works well to control infection, but it does have its unfortunate side—for example the violent immune response against foreign but harmless structures such as pollen grains, etc. (see Fig. 31).

Would-be parasitic micro-organisms that penetrate the barriers of skin or mucous membranes (top) have to run the gauntlet of four main recognition systems: complement (top right), **phagocytic cells** (centre), **antibody** (right), and **cell-mediated immunity** (bottom) together with their often inter-acting effector mechanisms. Unless primed by previous contact with the appropriate antigen, antibody and cell-mediated responses do not come into action for several days, whereas complement and phagocytic cells, being ever-present, act within minutes. There are also (top centre) specialized **natural** elements, such as lysozyme, interferon, etc., which act more or less non-specifically, much as **antibiotics** do.

Generally speaking, complement and antibody are most active against micro-organisms free in the blood or tissues, whilst cell-mediated responses are most active against those that seek refuge in cells (left). But which mechanism, if any, is actually effective, depends largely on the tactics of the micro-organism itself. Successful parasites are those able to evade, resist, or inhibit the relevant immune mechanisms, as illustrated in the following five figures.

Entry Many micro-organisms enter the body through wounds or bites, but others live on the skin or mucous membranes of the intestine, respiratory tract, etc., and are thus technically outside the body.

Surface barriers Skin and mucous membranes are to some extent protected by acid pH, enzymes, mucus, and other antimicrobial secretions.

Natural antibiotics Produced largely by macrophages, the antibacterial enzyme **lysozyme** (see Fig. 25) and the antiviral **interferons** (see Figs 22, 26), are responsible for a good deal of the natural immunity to what would otherwise be pathogenic organisms, and it is likely that other similar agents remain to be discovered, However, this type of protection is obviously restricted by the need to avoid damage to self material.

C3 Complement is activated directly ('alternative pathway') by many micro-organisms, leading to their lysis or phagocytosis. The same effect can also be achieved when C3 is activated by antibody ('classical pathway'; see Fig. 5).

T^H Helper T cell, responding to 'carrier' determinants and stimulating antibody synthesis by B cells. Viruses, bacteria, protozoa and worms have all been shown to function as fairly strong carriers, though there are a few organisms to which the antibody response appears to be T-independent.

B Antibody formation by B lymphocytes is an almost universal feature of infection, of great diagnostic as well as protective value. As a general rule, IgM antibodies come first, then IgG and the other classes; IgM is therefore often a sign of recent infection.

Blocking Where micro-organisms need to enter cells, antibody may block this by combining with their specific attachment site. Malaria and most viruses are examples. IgA in the intestine acts mainly in this way.

Phagocytosis by polymorphonuclear leucocytes or macrophages is the ultimate fate of most unsuccessful organisms. Both C3 and antibody tremendously improve this by attaching the microbe to the phagocytic cell through C3 or Fc receptors on the latter; this is known as 'opsonization' (see Fig. 8).

Intracellular killing Once inside the phagocytic cell, most organisms are killed and degraded by lysosomal enzymes. In certain cases, 'activation' of macrophages by T cells may be needed to trigger the killing process.

Extracellular killing Monocytes, polymorphs, and 'K' cells can kill antibody-coated cells *in vitro*, without phagocytosis; however, it is not clear how much this actually happens *in vivo*.

K 'Killer' cell, a lymphocyte-like (but not proved to be lymphoid) cell able to kill tumour cells extracellularly *in vitro*, through attachment of specific antibody to its receptors for the Fc region of IgG.

Intracellular survival Several important viruses, bacteria and protozoa can survive inside macrophages, where they resist killing. Other organisms survive within cells of muscle, liver, brain, etc. In such cases antibody cannot attack them and cell-mediated responses are the only hope.

T^C Cytotoxic T cell, specialized for killing, by lysis, 'self' cells altered by viruses, etc., and also allogeneic (e.g. grafted) cells (see Fig. 19).

T^H The helper cell of 'delayed hypersensitivity' which through its secreted cytokines attracts and activates monocytes, eosinophils, etc. (see Fig. 19).

Sequestration Micro-organisms which cannot be killed (e.g. some mycobacteria) or products which cannot be degraded (e.g. streptococcal cell walls) can be walled off by the formation of a granuloma by macrophages, often aided by cell-mediated immune responses (see Fig. 19).

Spread Successful micro-organisms must be able to leave the body and infect another one. Coughs and sneezes, faeces and insect bites are the commonest modes of spread.

Escape Some very successful parasites are able to escape all the above mentioned immunological destruction mechanisms by sophisticated protective devices of their own. Needless to say, these constitute some of the most chronic and intractable infectious diseases.

Inflammation Although some micro-organisms cause tissue damage directly (e.g. cytopathic viruses or the toxins of staphylococci), it is unfortunately true that much of the tissue damage resulting from infection is due to the response of the host. Acute and chronic inflammation are discussed in detail elsewhere (Figs 6, 34), but it is worth noting here that infectious organisms frequently place the host in a real dilemma: whether to eliminate the infection at all costs or to limit tissue damage and allow some of the organisms to survive. Given enough time, natural selection should arrive at the balance which is best for both parasite and host.

25 Immunity to bacteria

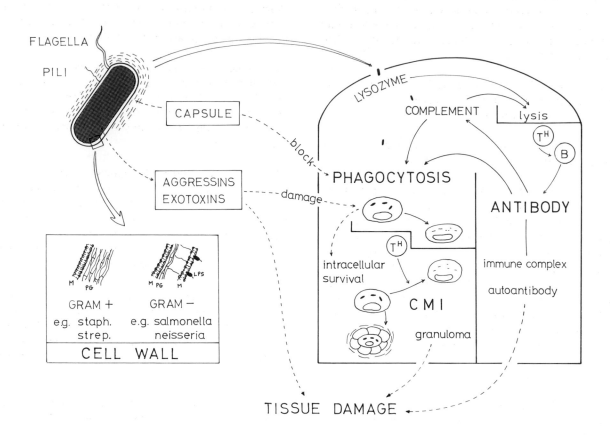

The usual destiny of unsuccessful bacteria is death by **phagocytosis;** survival therefore entails avoidance of this fate. The main ways in which a bacterium (top left) can achieve this lie in the **capsule** (affecting attachment), the **cell wall** (affecting digestion) and the release of **exotoxins** (which damage phagocytic and other cells). Fortunately most capsules and toxins are strongly antigenic and antibody overcomes many of their effects; this is the basis of the majority of anti-bacterial vaccines. In the figure, processes beneficial to the bacteria or harmful to the host are shown in broken lines.

Bacteria are prokaryocytes, unlike higher organisms from fungi to man (which are eukaryocytes) and this means that their structures and molecules are more foreign to us than fungi, protozoa, and worms; thus there is more chance of our evolving defences that attack the parasite and not the host. On the host side, the 'natural antibiotic' **lysozyme** represents perhaps the furthest point achieved in elaborating substances that attack bacteria but not host cells (until the antibiotic era; it is interesting that both lysozyme and penicillin were discovered by Sir Alexander Fleming).

Note that tissue damage may result from either the bacteria themselves or the host immune response. In the long run, no parasite that seriously damages or kills its host can count on its own survival, so that adaptation, which can be quite rapid in bacteria, usually tends to be in the direction of decreased virulence. But infections that are well adapted to their normal host can occasionally be highly virulent to man; plague (rats) and brucellosis (cattle) are examples of this ('zoonosis').

Cell wall Outside their plasma membrane (M in the figure) bacteria have a cell wall composed of a mucopeptide called peptidoglycan (PG); it is here that lysozyme acts by attacking the *N*-acetyl muramic acid–*N*-acetyl glucosamine links. In addition, Gram-negative bacteria have a second membrane with lipopolysaccharides (LPS, also called endotoxin) inserted in it.

Flagella, the main agent of bacterial motility, contain highly antigenic proteins (the 'H antigens' of typhoid, etc.) which give rise to immobilizing antibody.

Pili are used by bacteria to adhere to cells; antibody can prevent this (e.g. IgA against gonococcus).

Capsule Many bacteria owe their virulence to capsules, which protect them from contact with phagocytes. Most are large branched polysaccharide molecules, but some are protein. It is interesting that many of these capsular polysaccharides, and also some proteins from flagella, are T-independent antigens (see Fig. 17). Since T-independent antibody is thought to have preceded the T-dependent type in evolution (see Fig. 3), this fits in with the idea that bacteria were the main driving force for the development of the antibody-forming system. Examples of capsulated bacteria are pneumococcus, meningococcus and *Haemophilus*.

Exotoxins (as distinct from the **endotoxin** (LPS) of cell walls). Gram-positive bacteria often secrete proteins with destructive effects on phagocytes, local tissues, the CNS, etc.; frequently these are the cause of death. In addition there are proteins collectively known as **aggressins** which help the bacteria to spread by dissolving host tissue.

BACTERIA

In the figure, bacteria are given their popular rather than their proper taxonomic names. Some individual aspects of interest are listed below:

Strep *Streptococcus,* classified either by haemolytic exotoxins (α, β, γ) or cell wall antigens (groups A–Q). Group A, β-haemolytic are the most pathogenic, possessing capsules (M protein) that attach to mucous membranes but resist phagocytosis, numerous exotoxins (whence scarlet fever), indigestible cell walls causing severe cell-mediated reactions, antigens that cross-react with cardiac muscle (rheumatic fever), and a tendency to kidney-damaging immune complexes.

Staph *Staphylococcus.* Antiphagocytic factors include the fibrin-forming enzyme coagulase and protein A, which binds to the Fc portion of IgG, blocking opsonization, Numerous other toxins make staphylococci highly destructive, abscess-forming organisms.

Pneumococcus, meningococcus Typed by the polysaccharides of their capsules, and especially virulent in the tropics, where vaccines made from their capsular polysaccharides are proving highly effective in preventing epidemics. Patients with deficient antibody responses (see Fig. 38) are particularly prone to these infections.

Gonococcus IgA may block attachment to mucous surfaces, but the bacteria secrete a protease which destroys the IgA; thus the infection is seldom eliminated, leading to a 'carrier' state. Bacteria of this type are the only ones definitely shown to be disposed of by complement-mediated lysis.

Mycobacterium tuberculosis; leprosy These mycobacteria have very tough cell walls, rich in lipids, which resist intracellular killing; they can also inhibit phagosome-lysosome fusion. Chronic CMI results, with tissue destruction and scarring. In leprosy, a 'spectrum' between localization and dissemination corresponds to a predominance of CMI and of antibody respectively.

Shigella and **cholera** are confined to the intestine, and produce their effects by secreting exotoxins. However, antitoxin vaccines are much less effective than natural infection in inducing immunity, and attempts are being made to produce strains attenuated by genetic manipulations (see Fig. 40).

Salmonella (e.g. **S. typhi**) infects the intestine but can also survive and spread within macrophages.

Tetanus owes its severity to the rapid action of its exotoxin on the CNS. Antibody ('antitoxin') is highly effective at blocking toxin action—an example where neither complement nor phagocytic cells are needed.

Diphtheria also secretes powerful neurotoxins, but death can be due to local tissue damage in the larynx ('false membrane').

Syphilis should be mentioned as an example of bacteria surviving all forms of immune attack without sheltering inside cells. Autoantibody to mitochondrial cardiolipin is the basis of the Wasserman reaction. Cross-reactions of this type, due presumably to bacterial attempts to mimic host antigens and thus escape the attentions of the immune system, are clearly a problem to the host, who has to choose between ignoring the infection and making autoantibodies which may be damaging to his own tissues; see Fig. 35 for further discussion of autoimmunity.

Borrelia another spirochaete, has the property (found also with some viruses and protozoa) of varying its surface antigens to confuse the host's antibody-forming system. As a result, waves of infection are seen ('relapsing fever').

T^H Helper T cell, whose recognition of carrier determinants permits antibody responses by B cells and the activation of macrophages. There is little evidence that helper T cells ever react to absolutely unaltered 'self' antigens *in vivo* (but see Figs 21, 35).

B B lymphocyte, the potential antibody-forming cell. B lymphocytes that recognize many, though probably not all, 'self' determinants are found in normal animals; they can be switched on to make autoantibody by 'part-self' (or 'cross-reacting') antigens if a helper T cell can recognize a 'non-self' determinant on the same antigen (e.g. a drug or a virus; for further details see Fig. 35).

T^C Cytotoxic T cell, able to kill allogeneic or 'altered-self' targets. Cytotoxicity against 'pure' self may occur *in vitro* but has never been clearly shown *in vivo*, perhaps because it is so easily blocked.

Mast cell A tissue cell with basophilic granules containing vasoactive amines, etc., which can be released following interaction of antigen with passively acquired surface antibody (IgE), resulting in rapid inflammation—local ('allergy') or systemic ('anaphylaxis').

Complexes Combination with antigen is, of course, the basis of all effects of antibody. It is when the resulting complex is not phagocytosed, but instead circulates in 'soluble' form, that tissue damage may occur from the activation of complement, PMN, or platelets.

Complement is responsible for many of the tissue-damaging effects of antigen–antibody interactions, as well as their useful function against micro-organisms. The inflammatory effects are mostly due to the anaphylotoxins (C3a and C5a) which act on mast cells, while opsonization (by C3b) and lysis (by C5–9) are important in the destruction of transplanted cells and (via autoantibody) of auto-antigens.

PMN Polymorphonuclear leucocytes are attracted rapidly to sites of inflammation by complement-mediated chemotaxis, where they phagocytose antigen–antibody complexes; their lysosomal enzymes can cause tissue destruction, as in the classic Arthus reaction.

PL Platelets. Antigen–antibody complexes bind to and aggregate platelets, causing vascular obstruction as well as vasoactive amine release. Platelet aggregation is a prominent feature of kidney graft rejection.

MAC Macrophages are important in phagocytosis, but may also be attracted and activated, largely by T cells, to the site of antigen persistence, resulting in both tissue necrosis and granuloma formation. The slower arrival of monocytes and macrophages in the skin following antigen injection gave rise to the name 'delayed hypersensitivity'. Note that a number of microbial molecules can activate macrophages directly, for example the effect of bacterial endotoxin (**LPS**) in causing TNF and IL-1 release. When this occurs on a large scale, it can result in vascular collapse and damage to several organs. This 'endotoxin shock' is a feature of infections with meningococci and other Gram-negative bacteria. LPS can also directly activate the complement (alternative) and clotting pathways.

TYPES OF HYPERSENSITIVITY
(Gell and Coombs classification)

I Acute (anaphylactic; immediate; reaginic): mediated by IgE and sometimes IgG antibody together with mast cells (e.g. hay fever).

II Antibody-mediated (cytotoxic): mediated by IgG or IgM together with complement, K cells or phagocytic cells (e.g. blood transfusion reactions; many autoimmune diseases). It could be argued that this is not 'true' hypersensitivity, since these examples can be equally well classified as autoimmunity or transplant rejection, but see also V below.

III Complex-mediated: inflammation involving complement, polymorphs, etc. (e.g. Arthus reaction; serum sickness; chronic glomerulonephritis).

IV Cell-mediated (delayed; tuberculin-type): T cell dependent recruitment of macrophages, eosinophils, etc. (e.g. tuberculoid leprosy; schistosomal cirrhosis; viral skin rashes; skin graft rejection).

V Stimulatory: a recent proposal to split off from Type II those cases where antibody directly stimulates a cell function (e.g. stimulation of the thyroid TSH receptor in thyrotoxicosis). For the sake of completeness, a place must also be found somewhere for the 'blocking' and 'enhancing' antibodies of tumour immunity, and for polyclonal B cell activation (e.g. in trypanosomiasis), both of which can undoubtedly be against the patient's best interests.

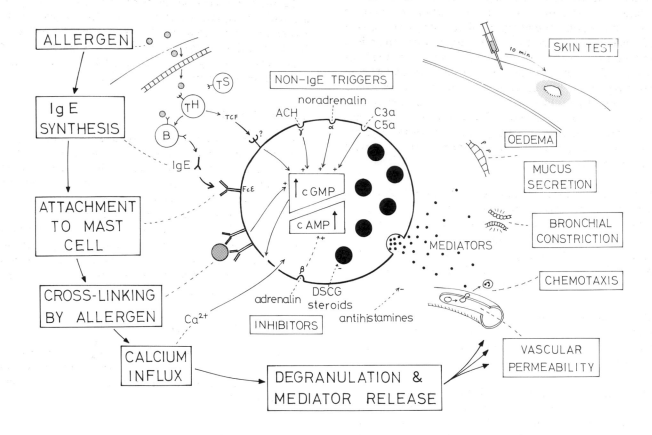

By far the commonest form of hypersensitivity is Gell and Coombs' Type I, which embraces such everyday **allergic** conditions as hay fever, eczema and urticaria but also the rare and terrifying **anaphylactic** reactions to bee stings, penicillin, etc. In both cases the underlying mechanism is a sudden degranulation of **mast cells** with the release of inflammatory **mediators**, triggered by specific antibodies of the **IgE** class. It is therefore an example of acute inflammation (as already described in Fig. 6) but induced by the presence of a particular antigen rather than by injury. With massive release (anaphylaxis) there is bronchospasm, vomiting, skin rashes, oedema of the nose and throat, and vascular collapse, sometimes fatal, whilst with more localized release one or other of these symptoms predominates, depending on the site of exposure to the antigen.

Antigens that can trigger these reactions are known as 'allergens'. People who suffer unduly from allergy are called 'atopic'; this trait is usually inherited and has been attributed to a variety of consitutional abnormalities. To justify the existence of this unpleasant and apparently useless form of immune response, it has been assumed to date from a time when worm infections were a serious evolutionary threat. Inflammation itself, of course, is an invaluable part of the response to injury and infection, and where injury is minimal (e.g. worms in the gut), IgE offers a rapid and specific trigger for increasing access of blood cells, etc., to the area.

There is a close link between inflammation and the emotions via the autonomic nervous system, through the influence of the sympathetic (α and β) and para-sympathetic (γ) receptors on intracellular levels of the cyclic nucleotides AMP and GMP, which in turn regulate cell function—in the case of mast cells, mediator release (see Fig. 23). Note also that mast cell degranulation can be triggered directly by tissue injury (see Fig. 6) and complement activation (see Fig. 33).

IgE The major class of reaginic (skin sensitizing; homo-cytotropic) antibody. Normally less than 1/10 000 of total Ig, its level can be up to 30 times higher, and specific antibody levels 100 times higher, in allergic or worm-infested patients. Binding of its Fc portion to receptors (Fcε) on mast cells and basophils, followed by cross-linking of adjacent molecules by antigen, triggers degranulation. Injection of antigen into the skin of allergic individuals causes inflammation within minutes—the 'immediate skin response'. Antigen responsiveness can be transferred to guinea-pigs by serum—the passive cutaneous anaphylaxis (PCA) test. IgG antibody by efficiently removing antigens, can protect against mast cell degranulation. However, some IgG subclasses (in the human, IgG4) may have transient reaginic effects as well.

T^H Helper T cell. IgE production by B cells is highly T cell dependent. There is also some evidence for a T cell derived factor (TCF) which binds to mast cells as IgE does. In atopic patients, allergens tend to induce the 'TH-2 type' cytokines IL4, IL5, etc. rather than, as in normal people, the 'TH-1' pattern (IFNγ). This is the best evidence so far that these T helper cell subsets exist in man.

T^S Suppressor T cell. IgE is also very sensitive to suppression, which may, together with IgG production, account for the success of 'desensitization' by specific antigen injections.

Mast cells in the tissues and blood **basophils** are broadly similar, but there are differences in the content of mediators. There are also important differences between the mast cells in the lung and gut ('mucosal') and those around blood vessels elsewhere ('connective tissue'). Mucosal mast cells are interesting in being regulated by (and according to some workers even derived from) T lymphocytes.

Ca^{2+} The entry of calcium ions is thought to be the first consequence of IgE cross-linking at the mast cell surface.

cAMP, cGMP cyclic adenosine/guanosine monophosphates, the relative levels of which regulate cell activity. A fall in the cAMP/cGMP ratio is favoured by Ca^{2+} entry and by activation of α and γ receptors, and results in degranulation. Activation of the β receptor (e.g. by adrenaline) has the opposite effect; atopic patients may have a partial defect of β receptor function, permitting excessive mediator release.

MEDIATORS

Many of these are preformed in the mast cell granules, including **histamine**, which increases vascular permeability and constricts bronchi, **chemotactic** factors for neutrophils and eosinophils, and a factor which activates platelets to release their own mediators. Others are newly formed after the mast cell is triggered, such as prostaglandins and leukotrienes (see Fig. 6 for details), which have similar effects to histamine but act less rapidly.

INHIBITORS

SCG Sodium chromoglycate ('Intal'), and **steriods** (e.g. betamethasone) are thought to inhibit mediator release by stabilizing lysosomal membranes. Other drugs used in allergy include **antihistamines** (which do not, however, counteract the other mediators), **adrenaline**, isoprenaline, etc., which stimulate β receptors, anti-cholinergics (e.g. atropine), which block γ receptors, and theophylline, which raises cAMP levels. It has been gratifying to physicians to see the new molecular pharmacology of cell regulation confirming so many of their empirical observations on the control of allergic disease.

NON-IgE TRIGGERING

The complement products C3a and C5a can cause mast cells to degranulate, and so can some chemicals and insect toxins. Such non-IgE mediated reactions are called 'anaphylactoid'.

ALLERGIC DISEASES

Originally the term 'atopy' referred only to hay fever and asthma, which are usually due to plant or animal 'allergens' in the air, such as pollens, fungi, and mites; it is still debatable whether all asthma is caused by allergy. However, similar allergens may also cause skin reactions (urticaria), either from local contact or following absorption. Urticaria after eating shellfish, strawberries, cow's milk, etc. is a clear case where the site of entry and the site of reaction are quite different, due to the ability of IgE antibodies to attach to mast cells anywhere in the body. There is mounting evidence for the role of food allergy in migraine and in other ill-defined physical and mental 'aches and pains'.

33 Immune complexes, complement and disease

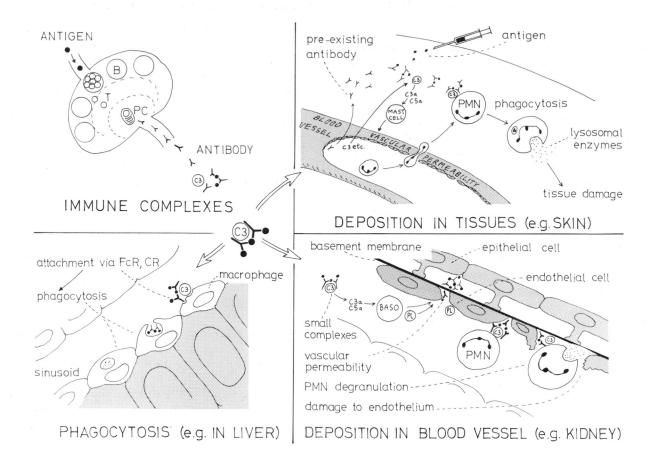

All the useful functions of antibody depend on its ability to combine with the corresponding antigen to form an **immune complex** (glance back at Fig. 18 to be reminded of the forces which bring this about). The normal fate of these complexes is phagocytosis (bottom left) which is greatly enhanced if complement becomes attached to the complex; thus complex formation is an essential prelude to antigen disposal.

However, there are circumstances when this fails to happen, particularly if the complexes are small (e.g. with proportions such as Ag2:Ab1; Ag3:Ab2). This can occur if there is an **excess** of antigen, as in persistent infections and in auto-immunity, or where the antibody is of very low affinity, or where there are defects of the phagocytic or the complement systems.

If not rapidly phagocytosed, complexes can induce serious inflammatory changes in either the tissues (top right) or in the walls of small blood vessels (bottom right), depending on the site of formation. In both cases it is activation of **complement** and enzyme release by **polymorphs** which do the damage, The renal glomerular capillaries are particularly vulnerable, and immune complex disease is the commonest cause of chronic glomerulonephritis, which is itself the most frequent cause of kidney failure.

Note that increased vascular permeability plays a pre-paratory role both for complex deposition in vessels and for exudation of complement and PMN into the tissues, underlining the close links between 'Type I' and 'Type III' hypersensitivity. Note also that complement activation on a large enough scale can cause acute widespread vascular damage, with both clotting and haemorrhage; this serious complication of bacterial and viral diseases is known by several imposing names (diffuse intravascular coagulation; massive complement activation; and, when caused by bacterial endotoxin, generalized Schwartzmann reaction).

Complexes of small size are formed in antigen excess, as occurs early in the antibody response to a large dose of antigen, or with persistent exposure due to drugs, chronic infections (e.g. streptococci, hepatitis, malaria), or associated with autoantibodies.

Macrophages lining the liver (Kupffer cells) or spleen sinusoids remove particles from the blood, including large complexes.

PMN Polymorphonuclear leucocyte, the principal phagocyte of blood, whose granules (lysosomes) contain numerous antibacterial enzymes. When these are released neighbouring cells are often damaged. This is particularly likely to happen when the PMN attempt to phagocytose complexes which are fixed to other tissues.

C3 The central component of complement, a series of serum proteins involved in inflammation and antibacterial immunity. C3 is split when complexes bind C1, C4 and C2, into a small fragment, C3a, which activates mast cells and basophils and a larger one, C3b, which promotes phagocytosis by attaching to receptors on PMN (and macrophages). Subsequent components generate chemotactic factors that attract PMN to the site. C3 can also be split via the 'alternative' pathway initiated by bacterial endotoxins, etc. Complement is also responsible for preventing the formation of large precipitates and solubilizing precipitates once they have formed (see also Fig. 5).

Mast cells, basophils, and **platelets** contribute to increased vascular permeability by releasing histamine, etc. (see Fig. 32).

The glomerular **basement membrane** (GBM), together with endothelial cell and external epithelial 'podocytes', separates blood from urine. Immune complexes are usually trapped on the blood side of the BM, except when antibody is directed specifically against the GBM itself (as in the autoimmune disease Goodpasture's syndrome) but small complexes can pass through the BM to accumulate in the urinary space. Mesangial cells may proliferate into the subendothelial space, presumably in an attempt to remove complexes. Endothelial proliferation may occur too, resulting in glomerular thickening and loss of function.

IMMUNE COMPLEX DISEASES

The classic types of immune complex disease, neither of which is much seen nowadays, are the **Arthus reaction**, in which antigen injected into the skin of animals with high levels of antibody induces local tissue necrosis (top right in figure) and **serum sickness**, in which passively injected serum, for example a horse antiserum used to treat pneumonia, induces an antibody response, early in the course of which small complexes are deposited in various blood vessels, causing a fever with skin and joint symptoms about a week later. Certain diseases, however, are thought to represent essentially the same type of pathological reactions.

SLE Systemic lupus erythematosus, a disease of unknown, possibly viral, origin in which autoantibodies to DNA and RNA are deposited, with complement, in the kidney, skin, joints, brain, etc. Treatment is by immunosuppression or, in severe cases, exchange transfusion to deplete autoantibody.

Polyarteritis nodosa; a disease of small arteries affecting numerous organs. Some cases may be due to complexes of hepatitis B antigen with antibody and complement.

RA Rheumatoid arthritis features both local (Arthustype) damage to joint surfaces and systemic vasculitis. The cause is unknown but autoantibodies to IgG are a constant finding.

Alveolitis caused by *Actinomyces* and other fungi (see Fig. 29) may be due to an Arthus-type reaction in the lung.

Thyroiditis and perhaps other autoimmune diseases may be due to complex-mediated (i.e. autoantigen plus autoantibody) damage to the organ. With developments in the technique of detecting immune complexes (there are now over 20 different methods, see Fig. 18) it is likely that more diseases will be added to this list.

34 Chronic and cell-mediated inflammation

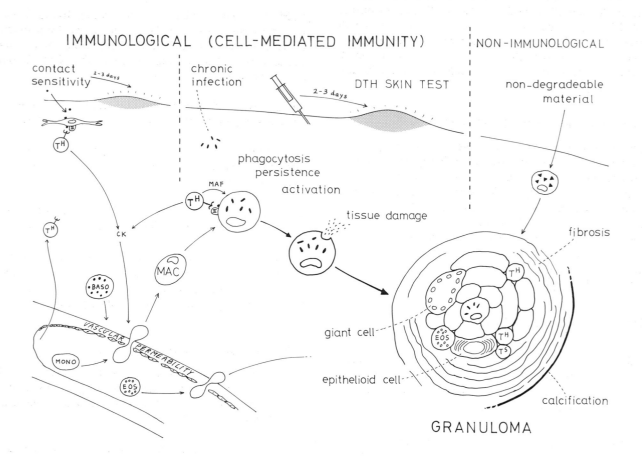

Following the changes in permeability, the activation of complement, and the influx of polymorphs, the last arrivals at sites of inflammation are the 'mononuclear cells': **lymphocytes** and **monocytes** (bottom left). Lymphocytes are usually specific in their attack, and only cause harm when attack is not called for (i.e. when the target is 'self' or a transplant), but monocytes and macrophages are equipped with enzymes which they normally use in the process of mopping up dead tissue cells and polymorphs, but which can also damage healthy cells, including other macrophages. When the stimulus is persistent, the result may be a growing mass of macrophages, or granuloma (bottom right), the hallmark of **chronic inflammation**.

These changes can occur in the absence of any specific immune response (e.g. reactions to foreign bodies; top right), but they are often greatly augmented by the activity of specific T lymphocytes (left) which, by secreting cyto-kines, attract and immobilize monocytes and activate macrophages. When this process is predominantly benefi-cial (as in healed tuberculosis) we speak of '**cell-mediated immunity**' (CMI); when it is harmful (as in contact sensi-tivity or schistosomal cirrhosis) it is termed '**Type IV hypersensitivity**', the underlying pathology being the same and the difference one of emphasis (compare with Fig. 19). Confusingly, direct killing by cytotoxic T cells is also called 'cell-mediated immunity', though since it mainly affects virus-containing cells, a better name would be 'cell-mediated autoimmunity' or, in the case of organ grafts, 'cell-mediated transplant rejection'.

In any case, it is rare for one type of tissue damage to occur in isolation, interaction of cells and sharing of biochemical pathways being a feature of immune mechanisms, useful and harmful alike.

CELL-MEDIATED IMMUNITY (CMI)

Contact between recirculating T cells and antigen leads to cytokine secretion with attraction and activation of monocytes and other myeloid cells (see Fig. 19 for further details). In the case of persistent antigens, particularly with intracellular infections such as tuberculosis, leprosy, brucellosis, leishmaniasis, schistosomiasis (the egg granuloma), trichinosis and fungi such as *Histoplasma*, chronic inflammation may result.

DELAYED HYPERSENSITIVITY (DTH)

The key feature of CMI is antigen-specific memory, which can be tested for *in vitro* by measuring lymphocyte proliferation or the release of cytokines such as IFNγ, or *in vivo* by the response to antigen injected into the skin. A positive DTH response consists of a reddened swelling 2–3 days later, the Mantoux test for tuberculosis being a typical example. While DTH frequently correlates with protective immunity, this is not invariably the case. Sometimes basophils are prominent, giving a quicker response known as 'Jones Mote' hypersensitivity.

CONTACT SENSITIVITY

In this variant of DTH, antigens (usually plant or chemical molecules) become attached to antigen-presenting Langerhans cells in the skin, where T^H cells respond to them. The result is an eczema-like reaction with oedema and mononuclear cell infiltration 1–2 days later.

CHRONIC NON-IMMUNOLOGICAL INFLAMMATION

Materials which are phagocytosed but cannot be degraded, or which are toxic to macrophages, such as talc, silica, asbestos, cotton wool, some metals and their salts and bacterial products such as the cell wall peptidoglycan of group A streptococci, will give rise to granulomas even in T cell deprived animals, and are therefore considered to be able to activate (or 'anger') macrophages without the aid of T cells.

GRANULOMAS

Granulomas are initiated and maintained by the recruitment of macrophages into the site where persistent antigen or toxic materials occur. Immune complexes are also a stimulus for granuloma formation.

Tissue damage may be caused by lysosomal enzymes released by macrophages, and perhaps by specialized cytotoxic molecules such as TNF (see Figs 30, 31).

Epithelioid cells are large cells found in palisades around necrotic tissue. They are thought to derive from macrophages, specialized for enzyme secretion rather than phagocytosis. There is some evidence that CMI favours their development.

Giant cells are formed by fusion of macrophages; they are particularly prominent in 'foreign-body' granulomas.

Eosinophils are often found in granulomas, perhaps attracted by antigen–antibody complexes, but also under the influence of T cells.

T^S T suppressor cells are thought in some cases to modulate granuloma formation by counteracting the T^H cells.

Fibrosis around a granuloma represents an attempt at 'healing'. Long-standing granulomas, i.e. healed tuberculosis, may eventually calcify, e.g. the well-known Ghon focus in the lung X-ray of many healthy people.

GRANULOMATOUS DISEASES

Apart from the known causes, granulomas are found in several diseases of unknown aetiology, suggesting an irritant or immunological origin. A few of the better-known are listed below:

Sarcoidosis is characterized by nodules in the lung, skin, eye, etc. An interesting feature is a profound deficiency of T cell immunity and often an increased Ig level and antibody responsiveness.

Crohn's disease (regional ileitis) is somewhat like sarcoidosis, but usually restricted to the intestine. It has been claimed that it is due to autoimmunity against gut antigens stimulated by cross-reacting bacteria. **Ulcerative colitis** may have a similar aetiology.

Temporal arteritis is a chronic inflammatory disease of arteries, with granulomas in which giant cells are prominent.

35 Autoimmunity

1	intracellular virus infection		pox, EB etc.
2	drugs, etc. attached to cells		sedormid penicillin malaria
3	cross-reacting antigens		group A β strep. spirochaete T. cruzi
4	cross-reacting idiotypes		?
5	late developing or sequestered antigens		lens, sperm
6	anomalous antigen presentation		thyroid, pancreas?
7	polyclonal activation		EB virus malaria, tryps adjuvants, GVH
8	deficient regulation	anti-idiotype networks	SLE ?

Autoimmunity is the mirror image of tolerance, reflecting the *loss* of tolerance to 'self', and before proceeding, the reader is recommended to glance back at Fig. 20, which summarizes the mechanisms by which the immune system normally safeguards its lymphocytes against self-reactivity.

These mechanisms can be overcome in a number of ways, and it is quite illusory to look for a single cause of autoimmunity. In the figure, eight possible ways are shown, and often two or more of these may occur together. Sometimes a 'self' cell displaying 'non-self' antigens is unavoidably destroyed in the process of eliminating the intruder (lines 1 and 2; foreign antigens are shown in black throughout the figure). Sometimes (lines 3 and 4) an invading organism sharing features with the host, triggers off an antibody response against normal 'self' (S). For this to happen there must be some self-reactive B cells already present (shown shaded in the figure); as explained in Fig. 20, clonal elimination of self-reactive cells is by no means complete, particularly for the B cells. Occasionally a 'self' antigen comes in contact with the immune system only at a late stage, when it is treated as 'non-self' (line 5).

Antigen presentation by cells not normally specialized for this role may give rise to self reactivity (line 6). Self-reactive B cells can be stimulated directly by 'polyclonal activators' which over-ride the usual triggering requirements (line 7). And finally, any breakdown in the suppressor cell and anti-idiotype regulatory networks (line 8) is likely to allow autoimmune reactions to build up to the point where they can cause disease. Note that the old idea that autoantibodies were simply new 'mutant' antibodies is out of fashion because they are so seldom monoclonal, although it may still apply in particular cases.

Understanding of autoimmunity has been advanced by animal experiments, in particular: (a) the induction of autoantibody in normal animals by cross-reacting ('part-self') antigens, assumed to be due to cooperation between self-reactive B and non-self-reactive T cells (line 3), and (b) spontaneous autoimmune diseases in inbred strains of animals, notably the NZB mouse and the OS chicken, which reveal a multiplicity of genetic influences, at the level of B cells, suppressor T cells, macrophages, target tissues, and hormones (autoimmunity is much commoner and more severe in females).

INDUCTION OF SELF-REACTIVITY

Viruses, especially those which bud from cells (see Figs 19, 26), become associated with MHC Class I antigens and the combination is recognized by cytotoxic T cells. Other viruses such as influenza may attach to red cells and induce autoantibody.

Drugs frequently bind to blood cells, either directly (e.g. sedormid to platelets; penicillin to red cells) or as complexes with antibody (e.g. quinidine). The case of α-methyl dopa is different in that the antibodies are against cell antigens, usually of the Rhesus blood group system, towards which B cell tolerance is particularly unstable.

Cross-reacting antigens shared between microbe and host may stimulate T help for otherwise silent self-reactive B cells—the 'T cell bypass'. Cardiac damage in streptococcal infections and Chagas' disease appear to be examples of this. With the development of computer 'banks' of protein sequences, a number of self-antigens have been found to share significant amino acid sequences with viruses and bacteria, suggesting that abnormal responses to infection may be an important trigger in many autoimmune diseases.

Cross-reacting idiotypes This idea is based on the demonstration of (1) idiotype-specific T helper cells, and (2) idiotype sharing between antibodies of different specificity. It might explain the autoantibodies seen during infections (e.g. mycoplasma) which do not react with the organism.

Late developing (e.g. sperm) or **sequestered** (e.g. lens protein) **antigens** are assumed not to be 'seen' by lymphocytes until released by organ damage (e.g. eye injury; mumps orchitis).

Anomalous antigen presentation may occur when, possibly as a result of virus infection, Class II antigens are expressed on normal tissue cells. Thyroiditis is the best studied example so far, and IFNγ is suspected of being one of the triggering factors.

Polyclonal activation Many microbial products, e.g. endotoxins, DNA, etc., can stimulate B cells, including self-reactive ones. The Epstein–Barr virus infects B cells themselves and can make them proliferate continuously.

Deficient regulation is easy to visualize but hard to prove. There is thought to be abnormally poor T suppressor function in SLE.

AUTOIMMUNE DISEASES

Autoantibodies are found in numerous conditions, often being clearly effect rather than cause (e.g. cardiolipin antibodies in syphilis). But in some diseases they are the first, major, or only detectable abnormality; some of the best-known are list below.

Haemolytic anaemia and **thrombocytopaenia,** though they can be due to drugs, are more often idiopathic. The correlation between autoantibody levels and cell destruction is not always very close, suggesting another pathological process at work.

Thyroiditis is one of the best candidates for 'primary' autoimmunity. There may be stimulation (thyrotoxicosis) by antibody against the receptor for pituitary TSH, or inhibition (myxoedema) by cell destruction, probably mediated by K cells and autoantibody. Anomalous expression of DR (HLA Class II) antigen is found in many cases.

Pernicious anaemia results from a deficiency of gastric intrinsic factor, the normal carrier for vitamin B12. This can be caused both by autoimmune destruction of the parietal cells (atrophic gastritis) and by autoantibodies to intrinsic factor itself.

Addison's disease (adrenal hypofunction), **diabetes**, and other endocrine diseases are often found together in patients or families with thyroid or gastric autoimmunity, suggesting an underlying genetic predisposition.

Myasthenia gravis, in which neuromuscular transmission is intermittently defective, is associated with autoantibodies to, and destruction of, the post-synaptic acetylcholine receptors. There are often thymic abnormalities and thymectomy may be curative, thought it is not really clear why.

Rheumatoid arthritis is characterized by, and may be due to, autoantibody against IgG, the joint damage being probably mediated via immune complexes. In this and other autoimmune diseases, the strong association with particular MHC antigens, especially at the D locus (DR3 and DR4 particularly), suggests that cell-surface recognition plays a basic initiating role; and abnormalities of the carbohydrate side chains of the Ig molecule also occur in this and some other diseases.

SLE In systemic lupus erythematosus the autoantibodies are against DNA and RNA, and the resulting immune complex deposition is widespread throughout the vascular system, giving rise to a 'non-organ-specific' pattern of disease. Like the 'organ specific' diseases (above), non-organ specific diseases tend to occur together. It is not clear why different complexes damage different organs; a localizing role for the antigen itself is an obvious possibility.

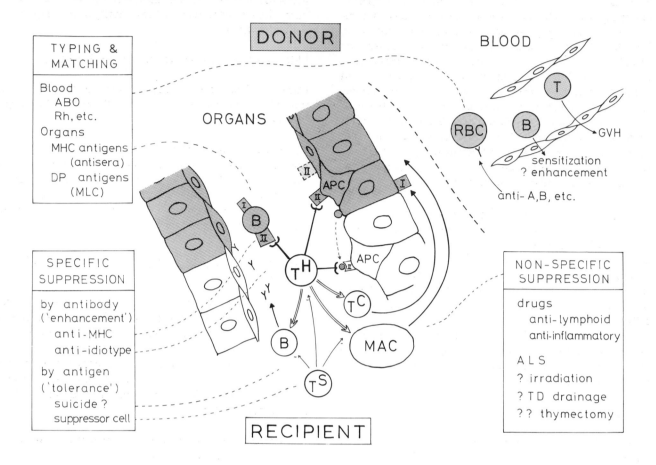

The success of organ grafts between identical ('syngenic'*) twins, and their rejection in all other cases, reflects the remarkable strength of immunological recognition of cell-surface antigens within a species. This is an unfortunate (and in the evolutionary sense unforeseeable) result of the specialization of T cells for detecting **alterations of MHC antigens**, upon which all adaptive responses depend (see Figs 17 and 19 for a reminder of the central role of T helper cells), plus the enormous degree of **MHC polymorphism** (different antigens in different individuals; see Fig. 13). It appears that when confronted with 'non-self' MHC molecules, T cells confuse them with 'self plus antigen', and in most cases probably 'self plus virus'; several clear examples of this have already been found in mouse experiments. This is probably the clue to MHC polymorphism itself: the more different varieties of 'self' a species contains, the less likely is any particular virus to pass undetected and decimate the whole species. Differences in red cell ('blood group') antigens also give trouble in blood transfusion (top right) because of antibody; here the rationale for polymorphism is less obvious, but it is much more restricted (e.g. six ABO phenotypes compared with over 10^4 for MHC). The 'minor' histocompatibility and blood-group antigens appear to be both less polymorphic and antigenically weaker.

Graft rejection can be mediated by T and/or B cells, with their usual non-specific effector adjuncts (complement, cytotoxic cells, macrophages, etc.), depending on the target: antibody destroys cells free in the blood, and reacts with vascular endothelium (e.g. of a grafted organ: centre) to initiate Type III inflammation, while T cells attack solid tissue directly or via macrophages (Type IV). Unless the recipient is already sensitized to donor antigens, these processes do not take effect for a week or more.

Successful organ grafting relies at present on (top left) matching donor and recipient MHC antigens as far as possible (relatives and especially siblings are more likely to share these), and (bottom right) suppressing the residual immune response. The ideal would be (bottom left) to induce specific unresponsiveness to MHC antigens, but this is still experimental (see Fig. 37).

* Terminology: *syn*genic, *syn*graft: between genetically identical individuals; *allo-* (formerly *homo-*) non-identical, within species; *xeno-* between species; *auto-* same individual.

TYPING AND MATCHING

For blood transfusion, the principle is simple: **A** and/or **B** antigens are detected by agglutination with specific antisera; this is always necessary because normal individuals have antibody against whichever antigen they lack. **Rh** (rhesus) antigens are also typed to avoid sensitizing women to those which a prospective child might carry, since Rh incompatibility can cause serious haemolytic disease in the foetus. Minor antigens only cause trouble in patients sensitized by repeated transfusions. Other possible consequences of blood transfusion are **sensitization** against MHC antigens carried on B cells, and, in severely immunodeficient patients, **GVH** (graft-versus-host) reactions by transfused T cells against host antigens. The latter is a major complication of bone-marrow grafting.

For organ (e.g. kidney) grafting, MHC antigens must be typed (as well as ABO). This is done in micro-cytotoxicity tests using B lymphocytes (the only conveniently obtainable cells that carry both Class I and Class II antigens), mono-specific antisera, and complement. The Class II antigens of the DP locus can only be typed by mixed lymphocyte reactions, a positive test being a stimulation of recipient T cells by donor B cells. The success of kidney grafting is related to the degree of match, particularly Class II (DR), but the better results with relatives suggest that there are other 'minor' histocompatibility loci so far undetected, as has been shown for the mouse.

REJECTION

The initial event is the recognition of 'altered self' Class II antigens by T helper cells. This can occur either by direct contact with donor B cells or antigen presenting cells (shaded APC in figure) or via the uptake of soluble donor antigens, (shaded circles) by the recipient's own APC. Following this, B cells, cytotoxic T cells and macrophages are all triggered into action; which response destroys the graft, depends on the organ in question. Some points of special interest are listed below:

Kidney graft rejection can be **immediate**, due to ABO mismatch or pre-existing anti HLA antibodies, **acute** (weeks to months) due to the immune response, or **chronic** (months to years) due to re-emergence of immune complex-mediated disease. Surprisingly, blood transfusion before grafting improves survival, perhaps by inducing enhancing antibodies against Class II donor antigens.

Bone marrow grafts are vigorously rejected, and require strong immunosuppresion. There is some evidence that NK cells may be involved. In addition, they can kill the host by GVH reaction, unless T cells are removed from the donor marrow.

Liver grafts are not so strongly rejected, and may even induce a degree of tolerance. HLA typing is less important.

Endocrine organs survive unexpectedly well if cultured or otherwise treated to remove the minority of cells expressing Class II antigens.

Skin grafts are rejected exclusively by T cells.

Cornea and **cartilage,** being non-vascular tissues, do not normally immunize the host and are allowed the 'privilege' of survival.

The normal **foetus** is of course an allograft, and why it is not rejected is still something of a mystery, despite evidence for a number of possible mechanisms, including specific suppressor cells, serum blocking and immunosuppressive factors, and special properties of both placenta (maternal) and trophoblast (foetal).

IMMUNOSUPPRESSION (see Fig. 37 for further details)

Non-specific suppression of lymphocyte division by cytotoxic drugs, together with the anti-inflammatory effects of steroids, are the mainstay of post-operative treatment.

ALS Anti-lymphocyte serum, sometimes used in the hope of avoiding damage to dividing non-lymphoid cells (bone marrow; gut). Nowadays monoclonal antibodies to the CD4 antigen are popular.

TD (thoracic duct) drainage and **thymectomy** are occasionally used to deplete T cells.

Irradiation Total-body X-irradiation is highly immunosuppressive, and local irradiation (e.g. of a kidney) or extracorporeal irradiation of blood to destroy lymphocytes, are sometimes used in acute rejection crises.

Specific suppression is directed at either the antigens inducing a response or the receptors on the cells carrying it out. When brought about by antibody, this is conventionally called **enhancement** and when by antigen, **tolerance**.

Suicide of specific T and B cells can be induced *in vitro* by letting them bind lethal (e.g. radioactive or drug-coupled) antigen.

Suppressor cells or antibodies, by mimicking normal 'network' control, might lead to stable tolerance, though this has not yet been achieved in man.

Landmarks in the history of immunology

1798   Jenner: vaccination against smallpox: the beginning of immunology.

1881–5   Pasteur: attenuated vaccines (cholera, anthrax, rabies).

1882   Metchnikoff: phagocytosis (in starfish).

1888   Roux; Yersin: diphtheria antitoxin (antibody).

1890   Von Behring: passive protection (tetanus) by antibody.

1891   Koch: delayed hypersensitivity (tuberculosis).

1893   Buchner: heat labile serum factor (complement).

1896   Widal: diagnosis by antibody (typhoid).

1897   Ehrlich: 'side chain' (receptor) theory.

1900   Landsteiner: ABO groups in blood transfusion.

1902   Portier & Richet: hypersensitivity.

1903   Arthus: local anaphylaxis.

1906   Von Pirquet: allergy.

1910   Dale: histamine.

1917–   Landsteiner: haptens, carriers and antibody specificity.

1922   Fleming: lysozyme.

1924   Glenny: adjuvants.

1936   Gorer: transplantation antigens.

1938   Tiselius & Kabat: antibodies as gammaglobulins.

1943   Chase: transfer of delayed hypersensitivity by cells.

1944–   Medawar: skin graft rejection as an immune response.

1945   Coombs: anti-globulin test for red-cell autoantibody.

1947   Owen: tolerance in cattle twins.

1952   Bruton: agammaglobulinaemia.

1953   Billingham, Brent & Medawar: neonatal induction of tolerance.

1956   Glick: bursa dependence of antibody response.

1956   Roitt & Doniach: autoantibodies in thyroid disease.

1957   Isaacs & Lindenman: interferon.

1959   Porter; Edelman: enzyme cleavage of antibody molecule.

1959   Gowans: lymphocyte recirculation.

1959   Burnet: clonal selection theory.

1960   Nowell: lymphocyte transformation (PHA).

1961–2   Miller; Good: thymus dependence of immune responses.

1966–7   Claman; Davies; Mitchison: T–B cell cooperation.

1971   Gershon: suppression by T cells.

1974   Jerne: network theory of immune regulation.

1975   Zinkernagel & Doherty; Bevan: dual recognition by T cells.

1975   Köhler & Milstein: monoclonal antibodies from hybridomas.

1980   Smallpox eradicated.

1981   AIDS recognized.

1984–   T cell receptor structure and genetics.

1987   Bjorkman: structure of MHC Class I molecule.

Some unsolved problems

AIDS: will a vaccine work?

Autoimmunity: is it all due to viruses?

Cancer: will immunology help?

Cytokines: (interleukins, interferons, growth factors): why so much overlap in function?

HLA and disease: how and why are they associated?

Human organ grafting: what are the critical antigens and will specific tolerance be possible?

Networks: how important are they in regulating immune responses and can they be exploited to control them?

T cells: do helpers and suppressors have the same repertoire? Do TH-1 and TH-2 subsets really exist?

Thymus hormones: are they real and will they be useful?

Transfer factor: what is it and how does it work?

Vaccination: will the parasite diseases succumb?

43 The CD classification

CD (cluster of differentiation) numbers are now used to identify **cell surface antigens** that can be distinguished by **monoclonal antibodies**. Some of these (e.g. CD25, 71) are clear-cut functional molecules, and several (e.g. CD3, 4, 8) are also widely used as **markers** of particular cell types.

A complete list is given below, with molecular weights and the major cell type on which they are found.

CD no.	MW	Cell type	CD no.	MW	Cell type
1	43–49 000	Thymocyte, APC	41	125 000	platelets
2	50 000	T, NK	42	145 000	platelets
3	16–25 000	T	43	95 000	T, myeloid
4	60 000	T helper, some mac	44	80–95 000	T, myeloid, rbc
5	57 000	some T, B	45	180–220 000	all leucocytes
6	120 000	T	45R	180–220 000	T subsets (? memory)
7	41 000	T, NK	46	56–66 000	all leucocytes
8	32 000	T cytotoxic	47	47–52 000	all leucocytes
9	24 000	pre-B, myeloid	48	41 000	all leucocytes
10	100 000	pre-B, leukaemia	49(a–f)	120–170 000	all leucocytes (adhesion)
11a	180 000	lymphoid, myeloid (adhesion molecules)	50	108–140 000	all leucocytes
11b	155 000		51	140 000	platelets
11c	150 000		52	28 000	leucocytes
12	90–120 000	myeloid	53	32–40 000	leucocytes
13	150 000	myeloid	54	90 000	act. T, B, mac (ICAM1)
14	55 000	mono, mac	55	70 000	leucocytes
15	(carbohydrate)	myeloid	56	135–220 000	NK, some T
16	50–65 000	myeloid, NK (FCR3)	57	110 000	NK
17	(lipid)	myeloid, platelet	58	40–65 000	leucocytes, rbc
18	95 000	as CD11	59	18–20 000	leucocytes, platelets
19	90 000	B	60	(glycolipid)	leucocytes, platelets
20	35 000	B	61	115 000	platelets
21	140 000	B (CR2)	62	140 000	platelets
22	135 000	B	63	53 000	platelets
23	45 000	B, myeloid (FCεR)	64	75 000	mono, mac (FCR1)
24	42 000	B, granulocyte	65	(glycolipid)	myeloid
25	55 000	act. T, B, mono (IL–2R)	66	180–200 000	granulocytes
26	120 000	T	67	100 000	granulocytes
27	110 000	T, some B	68	110 000	mac
28	44 000	some T	69	60 000	act. T, B
29	130 000	T, myeloid	70	?	act. T, B
30	105 000	act. T, B	71	190 000	proliferating cells (transferrin R)
31	140 000	mono, granulocyte	72	39/43 000	B
32	40 000	myeloid, B (FCR2)	73	69 000	B some T
33	67 000	myeloid	74	41/35/33 000	B, some mono
34	115 000	stem cells	75	53 000	B, some T
35	160–250 000	myeloid, B (CR1)	76	67–85 000	B, some T
36	90 000	mono, platelet	77	(glycolipid)	act. B
37	40–52 000	B	78	67 000	B
38	45 000	act. T, B, thymocyte			
39	80 000	B			
40	50 000	B			

act., activated; APC, antigen-presenting cell; CD, cluster of differentiation; CR, complement receptor; FCR, Fc receptor; ICAM, Intercellular adhesion molecule; IL-2R, IL-2 receptor; mac, macrophages; mono, monocyte; NK, natural killer.

Index

Page numbers in bold type indicate the figures on which principal references appear

ABO blood groups 36
Acute phase proteins 6
ADA deficiency 38
Adaptive immunity 1, 2
ADCC 9
Addison's disease 35
Adenoids 11
Adhesion molecules 14
Adjuvants 35, **40**
Adrenaline 32
Affinity **18**, 33
AFP 20, 30
Agammaglobulinaemia 38
Age, immunity and 38
Aggressins 25
AIDS 26, 38
Allelic exlusion 16
Allergy 32
Allograft 36
Allotype 16
Alternative pathway 5
Aluminium hydroxide 40
Amoeba 3, 27
Amphibians 3
Anaemia, haemolytic 35
Anaphylaxis 32
Anaphylotoxin 5, 6
Ankylosing spondylitis 13
Antibody 2
  deficiency 38
  diversity 15
  response 17
  structure 16
  undesirable effects 31
Antigen 2, 17
  division 30
  embryonic 30
  oral 20
  presentation 7, 17, 19
  sequestered 35
  suicide 20, 36, 37
  tumour specific 30
Antigenic variation 26, 27
Antihistamines 32
Anti-inflammatory drugs 32, 37
Antilymphocyte serum 37
Antiproliferative drugs 37
Apoptosis 10
Arthritis, rheumatoid 33, 35
Arthropods 3
Arthus reaction 33
Ascorbic acid 8
Aspergillus 29
Asthma 32
Ataxia telengectasia 38
Atopy; atopic 32
Autoantibody 25, 26, 27, **35**
Autoimmune disease 1, **35**
Avidity 18
Azathioprine 37

B, factor 5
B cell see B lymphocyte
B lymphocyte 9, 17
  activation, polyclonal 27
  deficiency 38

Babesia 27
Bacteria 25
BALT 11
Basement membrane 33
Basophil 4, 19, **32**
BCG 30, 40
Beta (β)2 microglobulin 13
Birds 3
Blast cell, transformation 4, 9
Blood transfusion 36
Bone marrow 4, 10
  grafting 36, 40
Borrelia 25
Bruton O.C. 38
Burkitt's lymphoma 30
Burnet F.M. 20
Bursa of Fabricius 10

C, 1–9 (complement) 5
C-reactive protein 6
Calcium 5, 32
Candidiasis 29
Capsule, bacterial 8, **25**
Carcino-embryonic antigen 30
Carrier 17
Catalase 8
Cathepsin 8
Cationic proteins 4, 8
Cell
  B 9
  K 9, 18, 24
  mast 2, 4, 6, **32**
  myeloid 4, 8
  NK 9, 30
  plasma 4, 9, 15
  stem 4
  T 9
Cell-mediated immunity 19
CGD 38
Chediak–Higashi disease 38
Chemotaxis 6
Chlorambucil 37
Chronic granulomatous disease 38
Class, immunoglobulin 16
Classical pathway 5
Clonal
  elimination 20, 37
  proliferation 17, 19
  selection 17, 19
Clone, hybrid 4
Clonorchis 28
Clotting, blood 6
Colony-stimulating factor 4
Combining site 16, 18
Complement 2, 5, 6, 33
  deficiencies 38
  receptors 5
Complex, immune **18**, 33
CON A 9
Concomitant immunity 28, 30
Constant region (Ig) 15, 16
Contact sensitivity 34
Coombs R.R.A. 31
Cooperation 2, 17
Copper 38
Corals 3

Corneal graft 36
Corynebacteria 40
Crohn's disease 34
Cross-reaction 35
Cryoprecipitation 18
Cryptosporidium 27
CSF 4, 22
Cyclic AMP, GMP 32
Cyclophosphamide 37
Cyclosporin A 37
Cyclostomes 3
Cytokines 22
Cytostasis 30
Cytotoxicity 19
  antibody-dependent 18

D, factor 5
Delayed hypersensitivity **19**, 30, 34
Dendritic cell 7
Determinant, antigenic 18
Dextran, dextran sulphate 9
Di George syndrome 38
Diabetes 35
Diffuse intravascular coagulation 33
Diphtheria 25
Domain, Ig 12, 16
Drugs, and autoimmunity 35
  and immunosuppression 37, 38
Dysgenesis, reticular 38

Echinoderms 3
Emotions 23, 32
Endoplasmic reticulum 8, 15
Endothelial cell 7
Endotoxic shock 31
Endotoxin 25, 33
Enhancement 20, 30, 37
Eosinophil 4, 8, 28
Epithelioid cell 19, 34
Epstein–Barr virus (EBV) 26
Exotoxin 25

Fab fragment of Ig 16
Factor B, D 5
Farmer's lung 29
Fasciola 28
Fc fragment of Ig 16
Feedback, antibody 17
Fibrosis 6, 34
Filaria 28
Fishes 3
Flagella 25
Foetal immunisation 20
  liver 10
Foetus, as graft 36
Food 20
Freund's adjuvant 40
Fungi 29

Gell P.G.H. 31
Gene,
  immunoglobulin 12, 13, **15**
  MHC receptor 12, 13
  T cell receptor 12, 14

Germ line   14, **15**
Germinal centre   11, 17
Giant cell   19, 34
Golgi apparatus   8
Grafting   36
Granulocyte   4
Granuloma   6, 19, **34**
Gut, lymphoid tissue   11
GVH (graft-versus-host)   36

Haemolytic anaemia   35
Haemopoiesis   4
Hagfish   3
Hapten   17
Hassal's corpuscle   10
Help   2, 17
Helper (T) cell   9, 17
Hepatitis virus   26, 33
Herpes virus   26
Histamine   6, 32
Histoplasmosis   29
HLA, H2   13
Hybrid clone   4
Hydrogen peroxide   8
Hydrophobic forces   8, 18
Hypersensitivity   1, **31**

I region   13
Idiotypes   21
Ig see Immunoglobulin
Immune adherence   7
Immune complex   **18**, 33
Immune response   1, 17, 19
Immunisation
   active   1, 40
   passive   40
Immunity   2
   cell mediated   19
   concomitant   28, 30
Immunodeficiency   38
Immunoglobulin (Ig)
   classes, etc.   16
   deficiency   38
   function   16, 18
   IgA   16, 25, 26
   IgD   16
   IgE   16, 28, 32
   IgG   16, 18
   IgM   16
Immunostimulation   30, **40**
Immunosuppression   26, 27, 37
Infection, immunity to   24–29
   opportunistic   27
Inflammation, acute   **6**, 32, 33
   chronic   34
Influenza   26
Insect bites   32
Interferon   2, 22, **26**, 30
Interleukins   19, 22
Iron   8, 38

J chain   16
J region   15
Jones–Mote hypersensitivity   34

K cell   9, 18, 24
KAF   5
Kappa chain   16
Kidney grafting   36
Killer T cell   19

Kupffer cell   7, 33
Kuru   26

Lactoferrin   8
LAF   19, 22
Lambda chain   16
Lamprey   3
Langerhans cell   7
Lectins   9
Leishmaniasis   27
Leprosy   25
Leukotrienes   6, 33
Light chain   16
Linkage disequilibrium   13
Lipopolysaccharide   9, 25
Liposome   40
Liver, foetal   10
LPS   9, 25
Lung   11
Ly antigens   9
Lymph node   11
Lymphocyte   2, **9**
   see also B lymphocyte, T lymphocyte
Lymphokines   19, 22
Lymphotoxin   19, 22, 30
Lysis   5, 18, 24
Lysosome   8, 9, 13
Lysozyme   2, 8, **25**
LyT antigens   9

M Protein   25
Macrophage   2, 7, 8, 17, 19, 20, 34
   activation   30, 40
Magnesium   5
Malaria   27
Malnutrition   38
MALT   11
Mantoux test   34
Marginal zone   11
Mast cell   2, 4, 6, **32**
Measles   26, 38, 40
Memory   2, 17, 19
Mesangium   7, 33
Metchnikoff E.   3
MHC   **13**, 36
Microfilament   8
Microglia   7
Micro-organisms, immunity to   24
Microtubule   8
MIF   19
Mixed lymphocyte reaction   36
Molluscs   3
Monoclonal antibody   9, 16
Monocyte   4, 6, 7, 34
Multiple sclerosis   26
Muramidase   2, 8, **25**
Mutation, somatic   **15**, 35
Myasthenia gravis   35
Mycobacteria   25
Mycoplasma   26
Myeloid cell   4, 8
Myeloma   16
Myeloperoxidase   8

Narcolepsy   13
Natural immunity   1, 2
NC cell   9
Networks   17, 20, 21
Nezelof syndrome   38
Niridazole   37
Nitric oxide   8
NK cell   2, 9, 30

Non-self   1, 20, 35
Nurse cells   10

Onchocerciasis   28
Oncogenes   26, 30
Opportunistic infection   27
Opsonization   **8**, 24
Osteoclast   7

Papain   16
Paracortex   11
PCA test   32
PEG   18
Pepsin   16
Peptidoglycan   25
Perforin   19
Permeability, vascular   **6**, 32
Pernicious anaemia   35
Peyer's patch   11
PHA   9
Phagocytosis   7, **8**
Phagosome   8
Pinocytosis   8
Plasma cell   4, 9, 15
Plasma exchange   37
Platelet   4, 6, 7, 31, 32
Pneumococcus   25
Pneumocystis   27, 29
PNP   9, 38
Pokeweed mitogen   9
Polio virus   26
Pollen   32
Polyarteritis nodosa   33
Poly-Ig receptor   12
Polymorph   4, 6, 7, 8, 31, 33
Polysaccharides   25, 40
Post-capillary venule   10
Pox virus   26
PPD   9
Pregnancy   36
Premunition   27
Presentation (antigen)   2, 7, 17, 19
Prion   26
Privileged sites (graft)   36
Properdin   5
Prostaglandins   6
Protozoa   3, 27

Qa antigens   13

Rabies vaccine   40
Reactive lysis   18
Reagin, reaginic antibody   32
Receptor
   Fc   8, 9, 32
   C3   8, 9
Relapsing fever   25
Replacement therapy   40
Reptiles   3
Restriction endonucleases   3
Retiarian therapy   37
Reticular cell   7
Reticular dysgenesis   38
Reticulo-endothelial system   7
Retroviruses   26, 30, 39
Rhesus blood groups   36
Rheumatoid arthritis   33, 35
Rickettsia   26
Ringworm   29
RNA, double-stranded   40
Rosette forming cell   9

Salmonella 25
Sarcoidosis 34
Schistosomiasis 28
Schwartzmann reaction 33
SCID 38
Secondary response 17, 19
Secretory piece 16
Self 1, 20, 35
Serotonin 32
Serum sickness 33
Severe combined immunodeficiency 38
Sequestered antigens 35
Sequestration 24, 34
Sharks 3
Shigella 25
Skin 11, 24, 29
SLE 33, 35
Smallpox 26, 40
Somatic mutation **15**, 35
Snakebite 40
Spleen 11
Sponges 3
Staphylococcus 25
Stem cell 4
Steroids 29, 37
Streptococcus 25, 34
Subclass (Ig) 16
Suicide, antigen 20, 36, 37
Superantigen 20
Superoxide 8
Suppressor T cell 9, 17, 20
Syngraft 36
Syphilis 25, 35

T3, T4, T8, T_i 14
T cell *see* T lymphocyte
T lymphocyte 9
 cytotoxic 9, 19
 helper 9, 17
 receptor **14**, 17, 19
 suppressor 9, 17, 20
 surveillance 30
Tapeworms 28
TCGF 19, 22
Temporal arteritis 33
Tetanus 25, 40
TGFβ 22
Theileria 27
Thrombocytopenia 35
Thy 1 (theta) 9, 12
Thymosin 4, **10**, 38
Thymus 10
 deficiency 38
 grafting 40
Thyroiditis 31, 33, 35
Tissue typing 36
TL antigen 9
Tolerance **20**, 37
Tonsil 11
Toxin 25
Toxoid 40
Toxoplasmosis 27
Trachoma 26
Transfer factor 29, 30, 40
Trypanosome 27
Tuberculin response 19
Tuberculosis 25

Tumour necrosis factor 22, 30
Tumours **30**, 38, 40
Tunicates 3
Typhoid 25
Typhus 26
Typing, tissue 36

UV light 11, 30

Vaccination 1, 21, **40**
Van der Waals forces 18
Variable region (Ig) 15, 16
Vascular permeability **6**, 32, 33, 34
Vasoamines 6, 32
Viruses, immunity to 26

Wiskott–Aldrich syndrome 38
Worms 3, 28

X-linked genes 38
X-rays 4, 36, 37
Xenograft 36

Yellow fever 26
Yolk sac 10

Zinc 38
Zoonoses 25, 26